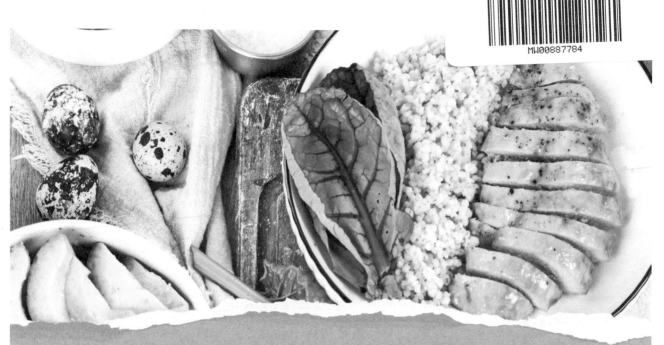

BY MARK RATOY

THE SUPER EASY
FATTY LIVER DIET COOKBOOK

2100+ Days of Healthy Recipes to a Leaner & Cleaner You:
Low-fat, Low-Carb Secrets to Smash NAFLD, Boost Detox, and
Accelerate Weight Loss | 28-day Meal Plan

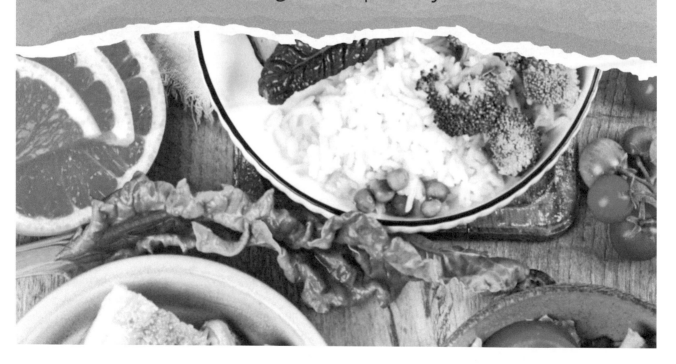

Disclaimer

This book is provided for educational and informational purposes only. It is not intended to replace professional medical advice, diagnosis, or treatment. Before beginning any new diet, exercise regimen, or treatment for fatty liver, it is essential to consult a qualified healthcare professional. This book's dietary approaches and information may only suit some individuals, as health conditions may vary.

The information presented is based on research and does not claim to be definitive or exhaustive. It is important to note that no guarantee is made regarding the complete accuracy or up-to-dateness of the information contained in the book. The authors and publishers bear no responsibility for any errors or omissions, nor for the outcomes derived from the use of this information.

The information provided in this book is to be used at the user's own risk. The authors and publishers expressly disclaim any liability of any type concerning any use, direct or indirect, of the information contained in this book.

Risk Acceptance and Responsibility

Purchasing or using this book implies acceptance of the fact that improving health through diet and lifestyle changes involves a process of experimentation. It is the individual's responsibility to evaluate their own physical and medical response to such changes. It is strongly advised to proceed under the supervision of qualified professionals.

4 BONUS

Find the QR Code on the last page to access your free bonuses!

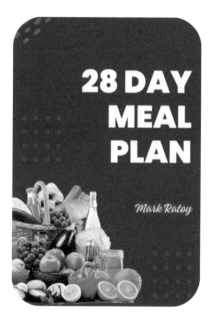

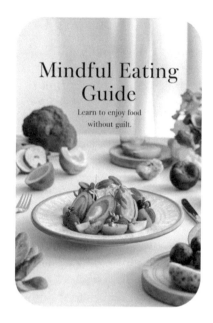

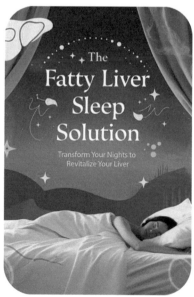

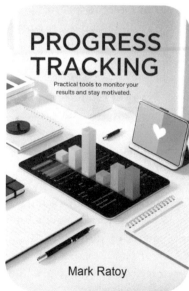

Table of Content

Why 2100 Days?

You might be wondering: with just 100 recipes, how can you create 2100 days of unique meal options? The secret lies in the power of combinations. Each recipe is a building block, and by combining them creatively, you can enjoy a new meal every day.

How It Works:

Breakfast: 20 recipes. Each recipe can be repeated once a month, providing variety for 20 days.

Lunch and Dinner: 40 recipes each. Alternating these recipes can create 800 unique combinations for lunch and dinner.

Mathematical Breakdown:

20 (breakfasts) x 800 (lunches) x 800 (dinners) = 12,800,000 unique combinations.

Even if you repeat combinations monthly, you still get 2100 days (about 5.7 years) of unique meals.

Key to Success:

Use flexibility and creativity to mix and match recipes.

Experiment with different combinations and flavors to find what works best for you.

With these 100 recipes, the possibilities are virtually endless. Start cooking and enjoy the journey to better liver health!

ABOUT THE AUTHOR

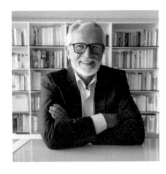

Dear Reader,

I welcome you to this journey toward understanding and managing fatty liver. I am Mark, a health and wellness enthusiast with a history of struggling with this condition.

My path began at a young age when I dreamed of becoming a doctor. I undertook medical studies at the University of Stanford. Still, after a year, I realized that that was not my path. However, my passion for health has never left me; in fact, it intensified when I faced the challenge of overweight and fatty liver firsthand.

I vividly remember the time when, during a fishing trip off the ocean coast, I experienced intense pain in my abdomen. Initially, I thought it was the usual fatigue from hours spent at sea, but the pain did not seem to subside as the days passed. After a series of tests, the diagnosis came: fatty liver.

Initially, I felt lost and bombarded with fragmented and biased information. But I took control of my health, delving deep into studying fatty liver and applying what I had learned to myself. With perseverance and determination, I witnessed remarkable results. My overall health improved, and my fatty liver regressed, even surprising my doctors.

For the past 15 years, I've been privileged to assist numerous individuals with fatty liver, sharing the knowledge I've gained. I've witnessed people regain their energy and vitality, shed excess weight, and enhance their health by implementing the methods I present in this guide. This rewarding experience has motivated me to write this comprehensive and scientifically sound tool for anyone struggling with this condition.

In the following few pages, I will share my experience and the latest scientific evidence presented in an accessible and practical way. I will guide you through the exploration of fatty liver, giving you the tools to recognize symptoms, understand test results, and take the necessary steps to maintain your liver health.

I want to be by your side on this journey, offering the knowledge and support you need to improve your condition and achieve your health goals. Together, we will work to make lasting changes in your lifestyle, step by step.

Remember, any progress counts, no matter how small. The important thing is to get started and not give up. You can make a difference in your liver health and life with the correct information and support.

I am excited to embark on this journey with you and look forward to sharing everything I have learned. I am honored to guide you on this journey to better liver health and a more fulfilling life.

With appreciation and dedication,

Mark Ratoy

Introduction to the VITAL Method

Welcome to the VITAL Method

Our body is an amazing machine, capable of regenerating itself and staying healthy when it receives the right nutrients. Although modern medicine offers many benefits, there is growing evidence that a natural, non-industrial diet can have a significant impact on our health, especially with regard to the liver. It is with this philosophy in mind that we developed the VITAL Method, a revolutionary approach based on scientifically proven principles and ancient traditions.

What is the VITAL Method?

The VITAL Method is an integrated system designed to support and improve liver health through five basic pillars:

V - Verify Dietary Habits.

The first step toward a healthy liver is to analyze your dietary habits. Verify what you eat on a daily basis and identify foods that could damage your liver. The VITAL Method helps you recognize these foods and replace them with healthier options that support liver function.

I - Integrate Natural Supplements.

The second pillar of the **VITAL Method** involves the supplementation of essential natural supplements. These include vitamins, minerals and other nutrients that support liver health. Supplements such as vitamins D, C, K2, Omega-3 and probiotics play a crucial role in keeping the liver in optimal condition.

T - Techniques for Detoxification.

Purification of the liver is a key element in maintaining its health. The **VITAL Method** introduces purification techniques based on specific foods known for their detox properties. By consuming a diet rich in fruits, vegetables and lean proteins, you can support your liver's natural detoxification process.

A - Active Lifestyle (Regular Physical Activity)

Regular physical activity is essential for good liver health. The **VITAL Method** includes a simple and practical exercise program that you can easily integrate into your daily routine. Physical activity improves blood circulation, supports liver cleansing, and helps maintain a healthy body weight.

L - Lifelong Healthy Habits.

Finally, the **VITAL Method** promotes the adoption of healthy and sustainable lifestyle habits. This includes stress management, adequate sleep and reducing exposure to environmental toxins. A holistic approach to health will not only improve your liver function but also contribute to your overall well-being.

How to Use the VITAL Method

In **"The Super Easy Fatty Liver Diet Cookbook,"** you will find a series of delicious and nutritious recipes, detailed food plans, and practical tips based on the **VITAL Method**. Each section of the book is designed to guide you step by step toward optimal liver health. Whether you are at the beginning of your liver health improvement journey or are looking to maintain your achievements, The **VITAL Method** will provide you with the tools you need to succeed.

Conclusion

The **VITAL Method** is not just a diet, but a lifestyle. By adopting these five basic pillars, you can significantly improve your liver health and enjoy a healthier, more energetic life. We invite you to discover the recipes, food plans, and practical tips that follow in this book and begin your journey to optimal liver health today.

Welcome to the VITAL Method!

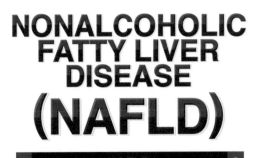

NONALCOHOLIC FATTY LIVER DISEASE (NAFLD)

| ○ | NAFLD | ○ |

is a condition in which excess fat builds up in the liver,
often related to obesity and insulin resistance,
which can lead to inflammation and scarring of the liver tissue.

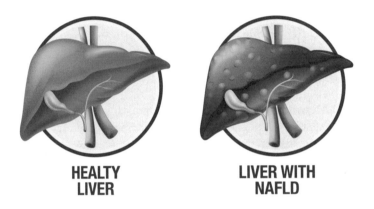

HEALTY LIVER **LIVER WITH NAFLD**

CHAPTER 1: WHAT IS FATTY LIVER?

1.1 Introduction

Greasy liver, too known as hepatic steatosis, is an progressively common condition caused by as well much fat collecting in liver cells. Envision your liver as a plant that works energetically to keep your body sound. When there's as well much fat, this manufacturing plant starts to slow down and not capacities effectively.

There are two fundamental sorts of greasy liver:

- **Nonalcoholic liver steatosis (NAFLD):** This is the most common form and is often related to factors such as obesity, type 2 diabetes, and metabolic syndrome.

- **Alcoholic liver steatosis (AFLD):** This form is caused by excessive alcohol consumption.

1.2 Why is Fatty Liver a Problem?

Within the early stages, greasy liver may not cause recognizable indications. In any case, on the off chance that not tended to, it can lead to more genuine issues such as:

- **Nonalcoholic steatohepatitis (NASH): A more serious frame of NAFLD including irritation and liver-cell harm.**

- **Fibrosis:** The formation of scar tissue within the liver can meddled with its work.

- **Cirrhosis:** An irreversible condition in which scar tissue replaces sound liver tissue, extremely compromising its work.

- **Liver cancer:** In uncommon cases, cirrhosis may increment the hazard of creating hepatocellular carcinoma (HCC). [1]

1.3 Risk and Development Factors

Several factors can increase the risk of developing fatty liver:

- **Obesity:** Excess weight, especially in the abdominal area, is a significant risk factor.

- **Type 2 diabetes:** Tall blood sugar can harm the liver.

- **Metabolic disorder:** A collection of conditions counting tall blood weight, tall cholesterol, and tall blood sugar.

- **Poor diet:** A diet high in saturated fats, refined sugars, and processed foods may contribute to fatty liver.

- **Need of physical movement:** An inactive way of life increases the chance of creating a greasy liver. [2]

- **Hereditary qualities:** A few individuals are hereditarily inclined to greasy liver.

- **Age:** The risk increases with age.

1.4 What Can You Do?

The great news is that greasy liver is frequently reversible with way of life changes. Within the taking after chapters, you'll learn how a adjusted slim down and physical action can assist you improve your liver wellbeing and anticipate complications.

Are you prepared to start your travel to a more advantageous liver? Perused on!

References

[1] Chalasani, N., et al. "The diagnosis and management of non-alcoholic fatty liver disease: Practice Guideline by the American Association for the Study of Liver Diseases, American College of Gastroenterology, and the American Gastroenterological Association." Hepatology 56.4 (2012): 1752-1766.

[2] Younossi, Z. M., et al. "Global burden of NAFLD and NASH: trends, predictions, risk factors and prevention." Nature Reviews Gastroenterology & Hepatology 15.1 (2018): 11-20.

CHAPTER 2: FATTY LIVER: DISTINGUISHING MYTH FROM REALITY.

2.1 Superfoods and Quick Cures: Myths and Realities.

One of the foremost determined myths concerns the adequacy of "superfoods" in treating greasy liver. Nourishments such as acai berries, turmeric, green tea, and coffee are regularly lauded for their antioxidant and anti-inflammatory properties. [1] Although these foods contain beneficial nutrients that can support overall health, it is essential to note that no single food can independently treat fatty liver.[2]

Fatty liver, or hepatic steatosis, is a multifaceted condition that requires a comprehensive, multidisciplinary approach. Effective management includes making significant lifestyle changes, adopting a balanced diet, engaging in regular physical activity, and, in some cases, implementing targeted medical interventions. Focusing solely on individual foods or supplements and neglecting other crucial aspects of disease management can lead to unsatisfactory outcomes and the progression of the condition.

It's crucial for individuals with fatty liver to consult with qualified health professionals, such as **hepatologists, nutritionists**, and **primary care physicians**. These professionals can develop a personalized treatment plan that takes into account the individual's unique needs. This plan should incorporate a balanced diet, regular physical activity, management of concurrent health conditions, and, if necessary, targeted drug therapies.

Instead of focusing on individual foods or supplements, adopting a **healthy and sustainable dietary** pattern, such as the **Mediterranean diet**, emphasizes consuming **whole foods, vegetables, fruits, healthy fats**, and **lean proteins** is more effective.[5] This nutritional approach, along with an active lifestyle and stress management, can promote liver health and promote overall well-being.

It's important to understand that there are no quick or miraculous solutions for **fatty liver**, despite the potential benefits of superfoods in a healthy diet. Effective management requires a sustained commitment to a **healthy lifestyle** and a multidisciplinary approach under the guidance of experienced health professionals.

2.2 Conventional Treatments: Limitations and Considerations.

Another common **misconception** concerns the effectiveness of conventional **drug treatments** for fatty liver. Antioxidants, **hypoglycemic agents,** and other treatments may be prescribed to manage specific symptoms or complications of NAFLD [7]. Although these drugs may help manage **inflammation** or **glucose metabolism**, it is important to note that they do not address the **underlying cause of** fat accumulation in the liver.[8]

The genuine control in overseeing greasy liver lies not in lessening liver fat levels alone, but moreover in progressing affront affectability, overseeing body weight and diminishing the hazard of cardiometabolic complications. This can be achieved through a **holistic**, multidisciplinary approach that goes beyond simple drug treatment. It's important for patients to understand that substantial **lifestyle** modifications, such as adopting a **healthy diet** and increasing **physical activity**, are often more effective than medication in the long-term management of fatty liver.

2.3 Diet and Weight Loss

Another widespread **misconception** is that only **drastic weight loss** can improve liver steatosis. Although weight reduction is undoubtedly beneficial, **how you lose weight** makes the difference. **Drastic diets** and excessive calorie restriction can actually worsen liver health in the long run.[11] It is far more beneficial to adopt a **balanced** diet high in **fiber**, low in **refined sugars** and **saturated fats**, and moderate in **calorie intake**.[12]

Opposite to well-known conviction, dispensing with fats from the slim down isn't the key to curing greasy liver. Our bodies require sound fats such as additional virgin olive oil, coconut oil, greasy angle, and berries. These advantageous fats offer assistance in decreasing systemic aggravation and bolster legitimate liver work. By understanding the significance of an adjusted eat-less diet, patients can make educated choices that engage them in their travels to oversee their greasy livers.

2.4 Toward a Deeper Understanding

Addressing common **myths** and **misconceptions** about fatty liver is a crucial step toward more effective management of this condition. **Education** and **awareness** can guide patients to avoid quick and ineffective solutions, encouraging them to adopt lifestyle modifications backed by solid **scientific evidence**.[15] An **informed** and **holistic** approach improves liver health and promotes long-term **overall well-being**.[16]

Through a greater understanding of the complexity of fatty liver and the factors contributing to its development and progression, patients and health professionals can work together to develop **individualized prevention** and **treatment strategies** that address each individual's specific challenges.[17] This path toward better awareness and informed action is essential to meaningfully address the **fatty liver epidemic** and improve the health and well-being of millions of people worldwide.[18]

References

[1] Petta, S., Gastaldelli, A., Rebelos, E., Bugianesi, E., Messa, P., Miele, L., ... & Bonino, F. (2016). Pathophysiology of nonalcoholic fatty liver disease. International journal of molecular sciences, 17(12), 2082.

[2] Rinella, M. E. (2015). Nonalcoholic fatty liver disease: a systematic review. Jama, 313(22), 2263-2273.

[3] El-Agroudy, N. N., Kurzbach, A., Rodionov, R. N., O'Sullivan, J., Roden, M., Birkenfeld, A. L., & Pesta, D. H. (2019). Are lifestyle therapies effective for NAFLD treatment?. Trends in Endocrinology & Metabolism, 30(10), 701-709.

[4] Alkhouri, N., & McCullough, A. J. (2012). Noninvasive diagnosis of NASH and liver fibrosis within the spectrum of NAFLD. Gastroenterology & hepatology, 8(10), 661.

[5] Zelber-Sagi, S., Solomon, F., & Mlynarsky, L. (2017). The Mediterranean dietary pattern as the diet of choice for non-alcoholic fatty liver disease: Evidence and plausible mechanisms. Liver International, 37(7), 936-949.

[6] Hannah, W. N., & Harrison, S. A. (2016). Lifestyle and dietary interventions in the management of nonalcoholic fatty liver disease. Digestive diseases and sciences, 61(5), 1365-1374.

[7] Sumida, Y., & Yoneda, M. (2018). Current and future pharmacological therapies for NAFLD/NASH. Journal of gastroenterology, 53(3), 362-376.

[8] Rotman, Y., & Sanyal, A. J. (2017). Current and upcoming pharmacotherapy for non-alcoholic fatty liver disease. Gut, 66(1), 180-190.

[9] Marchesini, G., Petta, S., & Dalle Grave, R. (2016). Diet, weight loss, and liver health in nonalcoholic fatty liver disease: Pathophysiology, evidence, and practice. Hepatology, 63(6), 2032-2043.

[10] Romero-Gómez, M., Zelber-Sagi, S., & Trenell, M. (2017). Treatment of NAFLD with diet, physical activity and exercise. Journal of hepatology, 67(4), 829-846.

[11] Johari, M. I., Yusoff, K., Haron, J., Nadarajan, C., Ibrahim, K. N., Wong, M. S., & Hafidz, M. I. A. (2019). A randomized controlled trial on the effectiveness and adherence of modified alternate-day calorie restriction in improving activity of non-alcoholic fatty liver disease. Scientific reports, 9(1), 1-11.

[12] Plaz Torres, M. C., Aghemo, A., Lleo, A., Bodini, G., Furnari, M., Marabotto, E., ... & Giannini, E. G. (2021). Mediterranean diet and NAFLD: what we know and questions that still need to be answered. Nutrients, 13(7), 2316.

[13] Yki-Järvinen, H. (2014). Non-alcoholic fatty liver disease as a cause and a consequence of metabolic syndrome. The Lancet Diabetes & endocrinology, 2(11), 901-910.

[14] Perdomo, C. M., Frühbeck, G., & Escalada, J. (2019). Impact of nutritional changes on nonalcoholic fatty liver disease. Nutrients, 11(3), 677.

[15] Chalasani, N., Younossi, Z., Lavine, J. E., Charlton, M., Cusi, K., Rinella, M., ... & Sanyal, A. J. (2018). The diagnosis and management of nonalcoholic fatty liver disease: practice guidance from the American Association for the Study of Liver Diseases. Hepatology, 67(1), 328-357.

[16] Kontogianni, M. D., & Tileli, N. (2021). The impact of Mediterranean diet on the development and management of non-alcoholic fatty liver disease (NAFLD). Metabolism, 123, 154920.

[17] Lazarus, J. V., Ekstedt, M., Marchesini, G., Mullen, J., Novak, K., Pericás, J. M., ... & Cortez-Pinto, H. (2020). A cross-sectional study of the public health response to non-alcoholic fatty liver disease in Europe. Journal of hepatology, 72(1), 14-24.

[18] Younossi, Z. M., Koenig, A. B., Abdelatif, D., Fazel, Y., Henry, L., & Wymer, M. (2016). Global epidemiology of nonalcoholic fatty liver disease-meta-analytic assessment of prevalence, incidence, and outcomes. Hepatology, 64(1), 73-84

CHAPTER 3: FUNDAMENTALS OF THE LIVER DIET FAT

3.1 The importance of a balanced diet for liver health

The liver, essential for metabolism and detoxification, can be compromised by unbalanced diets. Below is a summary of the primary nutrients and their sources:

- **Protein: Needed to repair liver cells; recommended sources include fish, poultry, and legumes.**

- **Healthy fats: Omega-3 and unsaturated fats found in foods such as avocados and fatty fish help reduce inflammation.**

- **Carbohydrates: Prefer whole grain sources such as quinoa and limit refined carbohydrates that contribute to fat accumulation in the liver.**

- **Vitamins and minerals: Nutrients such as vitamin E, vitamin C and magnesium support liver function.** [1]

3.1.1 Foods to avoid or limit

An inappropriate diet can contribute significantly to the development and progression of fatty liver. When consumed in excess, certain foods can increase **inflammation, oxidative stress,** and **fat accumulation in the liver.** To secure liver-wellbeing, it is significant to constrain or maintain a strategic distance from taking after nourishments:

Nourishments tall in soaked and trans fats: These undesirable fats are fundamentally found in greasy meats, matured cheeses, bundled prepared products, and browned nourishments. Soaked and trans fats can increment irritation and advance fat amassing in the liver. In any case, you can make a positive alter by choosing solid fat sources such as avocados, nuts, and vegetable oils like additional virgin olive oil, which can enhance your liver's wellbeing.

Foods high in saturated and trans fats	Healthier alternatives
Fatty meats (sausages, hamburgers, ribs)	Lean meats (chicken, turkey, lean beef)
Aged cheeses (parmesan, cheddar)	Low-fat cheeses (cottage cheese, mozzarella)
Packaged baked goods (cookies, cakes)	Fresh fruit, Greek yogurt with nuts
French fries, fried foods	Baked potatoes, steamed or grilled foods

High-glycemic-index foods: Foods such as white bread, white rice, potatoes, and sweets can cause rapid spikes in blood sugar, leading to an increase in **insulin** and promoting **fat storage in the liver.** Instead, choose low-glycemic-index **complex carbohydrates** such as brown rice, quinoa, and non-starchy vegetables.

Foods with a high glycemic index	Low glycemic index alternatives
White bread	Whole wheat bread, rye bread
White rice	Brown rice, quinoa
Potatoes	Sweet potatoes, pumpkin
Sweets, candies	Fresh fruit, berries

Sugary drinks and alcohol: Sugary drinks, including fruit juices and sodas, are high in **added sugars** that can contribute to **obesity** and **insulin resistance,** risk factors for fatty liver. Alcohol, when consumed in excess, can cause **inflammation** and **damage to liver cells.** Limit alcohol consumption and opt for unsweetened **water, tea** or **infusions.**

Beverage	Sugar content per 250 ml
Cola	27 g 0.95 oz
Orange juice	23 g 0.81 oz
Sweetened tea	22 g 0.78 oz
Water	0 g 0 oz
Unsweetened tea	0 g 0 oz

Processed and sodium-rich foods: Processed foods, such as packaged snacks, sauces and ready meals, are often high in **unhealthy fats**, **sugars** and **sodium.** Excess sodium can contribute to **high blood pressure** and **oxidative stress**, aggravating the condition of fatty liver. Instead, choose **whole** and fresh **foods**, and limit the use of high-sodium condiments.[2]

Processed foods with high sodium content	Healthier alternatives
Packaged snacks (chips, crackers)	Nuts, seeds, raw vegetables
Sauces (ketchup, mayonnaise)	Homemade tomato sauce, guacamole
Canned soups	Homemade soups with low-sodium broth
Frozen ready meals	Homemade meals using fresh ingredients

On your journey to reduce the consumption of these unhealthy foods, consider the following strategies:

- Scrutinized nourishment names and selected items moo in immersed fat, including sugar and sodium.

- Plan suppers at home using new, whole ingredients; you can control the quality and amount of ingredients.

- Maintain a strategic distance from browned or high-fat nourishments, vegetable dishes, inclined proteins, and sound fats when eating out.

- Discover solid options for your favorite nourishments, such as cauliflower-based pizzas or ice cream from frozen natural products.

Remember, the objective isn't to dispose of these nourishments but to restrain their utilization and energize more beneficial nourishment choices to bolster liver wellbeing. High-glycemic-index nourishments:Nourishments such as white bread, white rice, potatoes, and desserts can cause fast spikes in blood sugar, leading to an increment in affront and advancing fat capacity within the liver. Opt for low-glycemic-index complex carbohydrates like brown rice, quinoa, and non-starchy vegetables. These choices not only support your liver health but also provide a steady release of energy, keeping you feeling fuller for longer.

3.1.2 Key nutrients for liver health

A healthy liver diet should include:

- Omega-3 fatty acids reduce inflammation and are found in oily fish and flaxseed.

- Fiber: In fruits, vegetables, and whole grains, it aids digestion and toxin removal.[3]

3.1.3 Creating a liver-friendly eating plan

Now that we know the foods to limit and the critical nutrients for liver health let's combine everything and create a tasty and nutritious **eating plan** that will keep your liver happy. This is not about following a restrictive diet but making conscious, balanced choices that support long-term liver health.

Here are some practical tips for creating a liver-friendly eating plan:

Fill up on color: Fill your plate with a **rainbow** of fruits and vegetables. The more colors they include, the more **antioxidants**, **vitamins**, and **minerals you** provide your liver. Envision your plate as a palette of dynamic colors, with each color speaking to a wholesome superpower.

Select keen carbohydrates: Take complex carbohydrates, such as whole grains, legumes, and bland vegetables, rather than refined carbohydrates, such as white bread and pasta. Complex carbohydrates provide supported vitality and fiber that bolsters liver well-being. Think of them as your body's premium fuel.

Embrace healthy fats: Include **unsaturated fats** such as avocados, nuts, seeds, and vegetable oils in every meal. These healthy fats help **reduce inflammation** and promote liver health. Imagine sprinkling your meal with a bit of extra love for your liver.

Quality protein: Choose **lean** sources such as fish, poultry, eggs, and legumes. These foods provide essential **amino acids** for liver cell repair and regeneration. Think of protein as the tireless workers who work around the clock to keep your liver in top condition.

Plan meals:

1. Arrange your dinners and snacks a few times each week. This will help you make educated choices and have sound alternatives on hand.

2. Prepare extra meals to freeze for those busy days. This simple step can be a lifesaver, ensuring you always have a healthy, home-cooked meal ready, even when pressed for time.

3. Consider feast arranging as an act of adoring for yourself and your liver.

Remember that little, reliable changes over time can make an enormous difference in your liver's wellbeing. Celebrate each solid feast as a triumph, and be kind to yourself. With a top-notch and nutritious eating arrangement, you deliver your liver the adore and back its merits.

In the daily planning and recipe section, you'll find many practical and delicious ideas for putting these principles into practice in your daily routine. Read on to discover how to create tasty, liver-friendly meals and snacks that water your mouth!

We have investigated the fundamental standards of a liver-friendly count of calories; it is time to dig into the part of fundamental supplements in liver wellbeing. The following chapter will look at how particular vitamins, minerals, and other bioactive compounds back liver work and offer assistance in anticipating and overseeing greasy liver. Get prepared to jump into the lovely world of micronutrients and find their effect on your liver wellbeing.

References

[1] Zelber-Sagi, S., Solomon, F., & Mlynarsky, L. (2017). The Mediterranean dietary pattern as the diet of choice for non-alcoholic fatty liver disease: Evidence and plausible mechanisms. Liver International, 37(7), 936-949.

[2] Trovato, F. M., Catalano, D., Martines, G. F., Pace, P., &Trovato, G. M. (2015). Mediterranean diet and non-alcoholic fatty liver disease: The need for extended and comprehensive interventions. Clinical Nutrition, 34(1), 86-88.

[3] Gitto, S., Vitale, G., Villa, E., & Andreone, P. (2015). Treatment of nonalcoholic steatohepatitis in adults: Present and future. Gastroenterology Research and Practice, 2015, 732870.

CHAPTER 4: ESSENTIAL NUTRIENTS AND THEIR ROLE

4.1 Introduction to essential nutrients for liver health

The liver, essential to our well-being, requires various nutrients to function correctly. These include vitamins, minerals, and other bioactive compounds that protect the liver from damage and disease.

4.2 Essential vitamins for liver health

Vitamins are essential components of nutrition, continuously on standby to shield and support our liver. These crucial compounds are categorized into fat-soluble vitamins (A, D, E, K) and water-soluble vitamins (B, C). Each has a unique role in maintaining our liver's peak performance.

4.2.1 Fat-soluble vitamins (A, D, E, K)

- **Fat-soluble vitamins are the guardians of liver cell membranes. They break up into fats and can be put away in fat tissue when required. Here is a table summarizing their roles in liver health and the primary food sources:**

Vitamin	Role in liver health	Food sources
A	Supports liver cell regeneration and detoxification	Liver, eggs, carrots, spinach
D	Regulates calcium metabolism and supports immune function	Fatty fish, egg yolks, sun exposure
E	Powerful antioxidant that protects liver cells from oxidative damage	Nuts, seeds, vegetable oils, avocados
K	Essential for blood coagulation and bone health	Green leafy vegetables, broccoli, Brussels sprouts

To make sure you are getting enough **fat-soluble vitamins**, include a variety of foods rich in these nutrients in your diet. Remember, balance is key: too much of a good thing can be harmful; therefore, avoid overdoing it with supplements and focus on food sources.

4.2.2 Water-soluble vitamins (B, C)

Water-soluble vitamins are the queens of energy metabolism and detoxification. They dissolve in water, and our bodies eliminate the excess through urine, so we need to take them regularly in our diet. Here is a table summarizing their critical roles in liver health and the best food sources:

Vitamin	Role in liver health	Food sources
B (1, 2, 3, 5, 6, 7, 9, 12)	Support energy metabolism, detoxification and amino acid synthesis	Whole grains, legumes, green leafy vegetables, meat, fish
C	Powerful antioxidant that protects liver cells and supports collagen production	Citrus fruits, peppers, strawberries, kiwi, broccoli

To guarantee optimal intake of water-soluble vitamins, incorporate a variety of fruits, vegetables, whole grains, and sources of lean protein into your diet. These foods will provide essential vitamins, fiber, minerals, and other compounds beneficial to your liver.

Think of vitamins as essential nutrients, tirelessly working to protect and support your liver. By ensuring a steady supply of these vital nutrients through a balanced and varied diet, you're essentially arming your liver to face daily challenges and stay in top form.

4.3 Essential minerals for liver health

Minerals are the conductors of our metabolism, ensuring that every biological process is finely tuned. Essential nutrients can be divided into two categories: **macronutrients**, which we need in larger amounts, and **trace elements**, which are equally important but required in smaller amounts. Together, these minerals are crucial in maintaining our liver's health.

4.3.1 Macroelements (calcium, magnesium, potassium)

Macronutrients are the pillars of liver health, supporting several vital functions. Here may be a table summarizing their parts in liver wellbeing and the essential nourishment sources:

Mineral	Role in liver health	Food sources
Calcium	Regulates cell membrane permeability and supports inter-cellular communication	Dairy products, green leafy vegetables, sardines, tofu
Magnesium	Involved in more than 300 enzymatic reactions, including energy production and protein synthesis	Nuts, seeds, whole grains, legumes, green leafy vegetables
Potassium	Maintains cellular fluid balance and supports cardiovascular health	Bananas, sweet potatoes, spinach, avocado, beans

To ensure sufficient intake of these **macro-nutrients**, include a variety of whole foods such as fruits, vegetables, low-fat dairy products, nuts and seeds in your diet. A balanced diet will not only provide these essential minerals, but also several other nutrients beneficial to your liver.

4.3.2 Trace elements (iron, zinc, selenium)

Trace elements are the tireless workers behind the scenes, supporting a number of crucial liver functions. Here is a table highlighting their key roles and the best dietary sources:

Mineral	Role in liver health	Food sources
Iron	Essential for hemoglobin production and oxygen transport; involved in detoxification	Lean red meat, poultry, seafood, legumes, fortified cereals
Zinc	Supports immune function, protein synthesis and liver cell regeneration	Meat, seafood, nuts, seeds, legumes
Selenium	Powerful antioxidant that protects liver cells from oxidative damage	Brazil nuts, tuna, salmon, sunflower seeds, whole grains

To make sure you are getting enough **trace elements**, include a variety of animal and plant foods in your diet. Remember, small amounts of these minerals go a long way, so focus on quality rather than quantity.

Minerals are the silent superheroes that work tirelessly to keep your liver (and your whole body) in balance. By providing your body with these essential nutrients through a balanced and varied diet, you are giving your liver the tools it needs to function at its best and support your overall health.

In the next section, we will explore the fascinating world of bioactive compounds and discover how these phytochemical superheroes can transform your liver health!

4.4 Other bioactive compounds for liver health

In addition to essential vitamins and minerals, another group of nutritional superheroes deserves our recognition: **bio-**

active compounds. These powerful phytochemicals, found naturally in plants, have incredible effects on liver health, from reducing inflammation to protecting against oxidative damage.

4.4.1 Antioxidants (polyphenols, flavonoids)

Antioxidants, the champions of detoxification, stand ready to neutralize harmful free radicals that can harm liver cells. Among these, polyphenols and flavonoids are **two** powerful **groups**. A comprehensive table detailing their action mechanisms and the top food sources is provided below:

Antioxidant	Mechanism of action	Food sources
Polyphenols	Neutralize free radicals, reduce inflammation and support detoxification	Green tea, turmeric, berries, cocoa, olives
Flavonoids	They protect liver cells from oxidative damage, improve insulin sensitivity and support immune function	Fruits, vegetables, herbs, spices, tea, dark chocolate

To harness the power of antioxidants, include a variety of colorful plant foods in your diet. The more colors you add to your plate, the wider the range of bioactive compounds you will provide to your liver.

4.4.2 Essential fatty acids (omega-3, omega-6)

Essential fatty acids, particularly **omega-3** and **omega-6**, are the guardians of liver cell membrane health. These beneficial fats are crucial in regulating inflammation and supporting overall liver function. Here is a table highlighting their roles and the best dietary sources:

Fatty acid	Role in liver health	Food sources
Omega-3	Reduce inflammation, improve insulin sensitivity and support cardiovascular health	Fatty fish (salmon, sardines, mackerel), nuts, flaxseeds, chia seeds
Omega-6	Support immune function and cell membrane health	Vegetable oils (sunflower, safflower, corn), nuts, seeds

High quality of both omega-3 and omega-6. Remember, balance is critical: an unbalanced ratio of omega-6 to omega-3 can contribute to inflammation, so focus on increasing your intake of omega-3-rich foods.

Bioactive compounds are the silent superheroes working tirelessly to protect and support your liver's health. Including various colorful plant foods and high-quality sources of essential fatty acids in your diet gives your liver the tools to thrive and support your overall well-being.

The following section will explore the fascinating interactions between various nutrients and discover how a balanced and varied diet can transform your liver health!

4.5 The Interplay of Nutrients and Liver Health

Envision your body as an intricate symphony, where each nutrient plays a vital role in creating a harmony of health and well-being. Much like an orchestra, the various nutrients do not function in isolation but interact and complement each other to support the health of the liver and the entire body.

Vitamins, minerals, and **bioactive compounds** are the musicians in this nutrient symphony, each with its unique but interconnected role. For example:

- **Vitamin C enhances iron absorption, promoting hemoglobin production and oxygen transportation.**

- **Vitamin D works in synergy with calcium to maintain bone health and support immune function.**

- **Polyphenols and flavonoids collaborate to neutralize free radicals and reduce inflammation, fostering an environment conducive to liver health.**

These are just a few nutrient interactions contributing to liver and body health.

Moreover, it's crucial to understand that you hold power regarding your liver health. No single food or nutrient is a magic wand for liver health. Instead, the symphony of a **balanced and varied diet** creates the optimal conditions for liver wellness. Consider it a nutritional smorgasbord: the more colors, flavors, and textures you add to your plate, the more comprehensive the range of beneficial nutrients you provide to your liver. This knowledge empowers you to make informed choices and take charge of your liver's health.

Ultimately, your liver is the maestro of your metabolism, tirelessly working to keep your body in balance. Understanding the role of various nutrients and their interactions is the first step in creating a nutritional symphony that supports your liver's health. In the following sections, we will delve into practical strategies and delicious recipes that will help you put this knowledge into practice and give your liver the nourishment it needs to thrive. Remember, a healthy liver is not just about liver health but about overall well-being.

Remember, every bite you put on your plate is an opportunity to nourish and pamper your liver. With the information presented in this chapter as a foundation, you are now equipped to embark on an exciting journey toward a healthier liver and optimal overall wellness. Turning the page, you will discover how to turn this knowledge into action and create a personalized roadmap for your liver health. The future is bright, and your liver looks forward to accompanying you on this journey. Rest assured, the strategies and recipes we will explore are simple, practical, and delicious, making your liver health journey joyous.

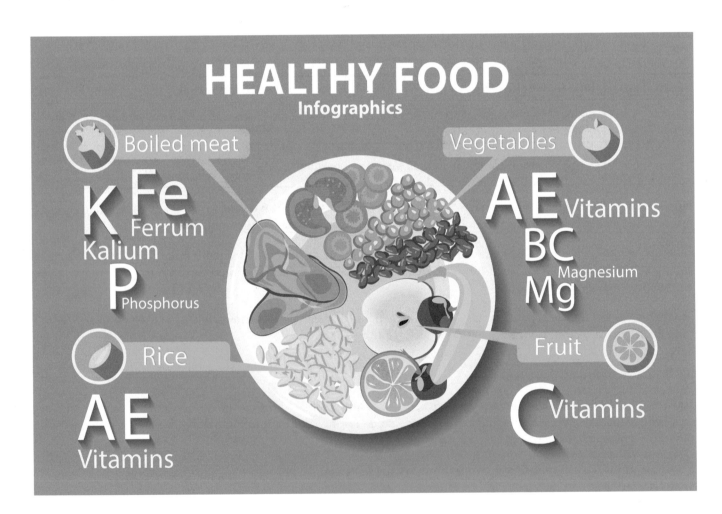

CHAPTER 5: OTHER WAYS TO IMPROVE LIVER HEALTH

5.1 Introduction to Complementary Strategies

In addition to diet, regular exercise and stress management are not just beneficial. Still, they also put you in the driver's seat of your liver health. Physical activity helps improve insulin sensitivity and reduce inflammation. At the same time, relaxation techniques such as meditation and yoga can empower you to mitigate the impact of chronic stress on the liver. [1] It is also crucial to maintain a healthy weight to prevent disorders such as nonalcoholic hepatic steatosis (NAFLD).

5.2 Importance of Physical Exercise

Exercise controls weight, improves insulin sensitivity, and promotes circulation, benefiting liver function. Even moderate physical activity, such as walking for 30 minutes daily, can significantly and positively affect liver health, giving you hope for a healthier liver.

5.3 Stress Management and Relaxation

Stress reduction is essential for liver health, as chronic stress can exacerbate inflammation and impair detoxification. Mindfulness practices and yoga reduce stress and improve liver function through improved circulation and digestion.[2]

5.4 Body Weight Control

A healthy body weight is critical to preventing NAFLD. Strategies for maintaining or achieving an ideal weight include a balanced diet rich in whole foods and a regular exercise routine. Even modest weight loss can significantly improve hepatic steatosis and reduce inflammation.[3]

References

[1] Chacko, K. R., & Reinus, J. (2016). Extrahepatic complications of nonalcoholic fatty liver disease. Clinics in Liver Disease, 20(2), 387-401.

[2] Korman, J. B., & Volenberg, I. (2018). Complementary and alternative medicine approaches to the treatment of nonalcoholic fatty liver disease. In Non-Alcoholic fatty liver disease (pp. 315-331). Springer, Cham.

[3] Hannah, W. N., & Harrison, S. A. (2016). Effect of weight loss, diet, exercise, and bariatric surgery on nonalcoholic fatty liver disease. Clinics in Liver Disease, 20(2), 339-350.

CHAPTER 6: MEAL PLANNING AND SHOPPING LIST

6.1 Introduction to the importance of meal planning

Meal planning is not just a helpful tool; it's a crucial strategy in managing fatty liver. When planned in advance, a well-structured diet can significantly promote liver health and encourage weight loss, a key factor in reducing hepatic steatosis. By planning your meals, you gain the power to make more informed food choices, steer clear of unhealthy temptations, and even save time and money.

6.2 Basic principles for effective planning

6.2.1 Consider specific nutritional needs for fatty liver

It is essential to incorporate fiber- and nutrient-rich foods, limit saturated fats and sugars, and include healthy fats such as omega-3s.

6.2.2 Variety and balance of nutrients

It is essential to ensure variety and balance to get nutrients and keep meals interesting. A straightforward way is to follow the "healthy plate" model in every main meal:

- **1/2 dish: non-starchy vegetable**

- **1/4 plate: lean protein**

- **1/4 plate: complex carbohydrates**

- **A punch: healthy fats**

6.2.3 Adequate portions

Controlling portions is crucial for weight and fatty liver management. Here are some general guidelines:

Food	Portion
Non-starchy vegetables	1 cup raw (250 ml), 1/2 cup cooked (125 ml)
Fruit	1 medium piece, 1 piece cup (250 ml)
Lean protein	Palm size (85-110g / 3-4 oz)
Complex carbohydrates	1/2 cup cooked (125 ml) (pasta, rice, cereal)
Healthy fats	1 tablespoon (15 ml) (oil, seed, avocado)

6.2.4 Personal preferences and lifestyle

Adapt planning to your personal taste, considering your routine and available budget.

6.3 Creating a weekly meal plan

6.3.1 Sample outline of a weekly plan

Day	Breakfast	Lunch	Dinner	Snack
Monday	Greek yogurt with walnuts and blueberries	Quinoa salad with chickpeas and mixed vegetables	Baked salmon with asparagus and sweet potatoes	Almonds and an apple
Tuesday	Spinach and banana smoothie	Lentil soup with whole wheat bread	Grilled chicken breast with broccoli	Greek yogurt and honey
Wednesday	Oats with apples and cinnamon	Tuna salad with avocado	Tofu stir-fry with mixed vegetables and quinoa	Carrots and hummus
Thursday	Spinach and mushroom omelette	Chicken wrap with hummus and vegetables	Baked cod with spinach and roasted potatoes	Orange slices
Friday	Oatmeal pancakes with raspberries	Greek salad with chicken	Lean porterhouse steak with arugula salad	Dried fruit mix
Saturday	Smoothie bowl with berries and chia	Burrito bowl with brown rice and black beans	Zucchini spaghetti with turkey meatballs	Vegetable chips
Sunday	Poached eggs with spinach and avocado	Beet salad with walnuts and goat cheese	Roast pork with carrots and coleslaw	Dark chocolate and nuts

Note: Selected ingredients are readily available and inexpensive in both the United States and the United Kingdom.

6.3.2 Tips for preparing meals in advance

- Dedicate a couple of hours on the weekend to prepare essential ingredients (rice, cooked protein, cut vegetables)

- Uses "batch cooking" technique to cook extra portions for freezing.

- Make creative use of leftovers for later meals.

- Keep healthy, ready-to-use foods on hand at all times.

6.3.3 Strategies for managing meals outside the home

- Study the restaurant menu in advance and make informed choices.

- Ask for changes (e.g., steamed vegetables instead of fried)

- Control portions (e.g., ask to pack half a plate to take home)

- Balance more elaborate meals with light options for the rest of the day.

6.4 Shopping list

6.4.1 Organizing your shopping List by meal plan

Once you have created your weekly meal plan, prepare a shopping list organized by:

- **Meals (breakfast, lunch, dinner, snacks)**

- **Food categories (fruits, vegetables, protein, dairy, pantry)**

This will help you to be efficient at the supermarket and remember critical ingredients.

6.4.2 Tips for intelligent and conscious spending

- **Don't shop when you're hungry to avoid impulse purchases.**

- **Choose seasonal and local produce (cheaper and more nutritious)**

- **Compare prices and opt for supermarket brands whenever possible.**

- **Read nutrition labels (look for low saturated fat, sugar, and sodium)**

6.4.3 Focus on inexpensive and accessible hepatoprotective foods

When compiling your shopping list, prioritize foods that promote liver health that are readily available and inexpensive:

- **Green leafy vegetables (spinach, kale, lettuce)**

- **Cheap crucifers (cabbage, cauliflower, broccoli)**

- **Fruits rich in antioxidants (apples, oranges, bananas)**

- **Vegetable protein (beans, lentils, chickpeas)**

- **Cheap whole grains (oats, brown rice, whole wheat pasta)**

- **Cheap healthy fats (coconut oil, flaxseed, natural peanut butter)**

- **Antioxidant spices and herbs (turmeric, oregano, basil)**

Regularly including these affordable foods in your grocery shopping will help you create balanced meals that benefit your liver without straining your wallet.

Meal planning and mindful spending are skills that take practice, but the benefits to your liver health are worth the effort. Start gradually, be flexible and find the strategies that work best for you. Over time, this process will become a natural healthy habit.

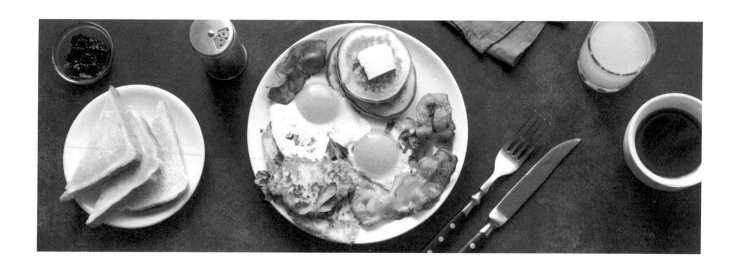

CHAPTER 7: HEALTHY AND TASTY BREAKFAST RECIPES

7.1 Importance of a balanced breakfast

Breakfast is often considered the most important meal and with good reason. After fasting overnight, our bodies need to replenish themselves with energy and nutrients to better cope with daily activities. A balanced and healthy breakfast is even more crucial for those suffering from liver fatty liver, as it can help improve liver health and support detoxification.

Skipping breakfast or consuming low-nutrient, high-sugar, or high-fat foods can lead to glycemic spikes, fatiguing the liver and promoting fat accumulation in the organ. In contrast, a balanced breakfast of complex carbohydrates, lean protein, good fats, and fiber gradually releases energy, stabilizes blood sugar levels, and promotes satiety, reducing the risk of binge eating or poor food choices during the rest of the day.

In addition, eating a healthy breakfast helps to awaken the metabolism, stimulate digestive processes, and promote fat burning. This is especially beneficial for those suffering from fatty liver, as an efficient metabolism facilitates the mobilization and elimination of excess fat deposits, including in the liver.

But what makes a genuinely balanced breakfast? An ideal mix should include:

1. Complex carbohydrates, such as whole grains, whole grain breads, oats, and quinoa, provide slow-release energy and fiber that promote intestinal regularity.

2. Lean proteins, such as eggs, Greek yogurt, cottage cheese, tofu, or salmon, help preserve muscle mass, promote satiety, and support cellular repair.

3. Good fats: avocados, nuts, seeds, and olive oil provide essential fatty acids and fat-soluble vitamins and support cardiovascular health.

4. Fruits and vegetables provide vitamins, minerals, antioxidants, and fiber, protecting the liver from oxidative stress and promoting detoxification.

5. Healthy drinks: water, green tea, and sugar-free coffee help hydrate the body and stimulate digestive functions.

In the following few pages, you will find many tasty and balanced breakfast recipes specifically designed to support your liver health without sacrificing your enjoyment of food. You will learn how to combine the right ingredients to start your day with energy, taste, and vitality, which will benefit your liver and body.

Egg-white omelet with vegetables

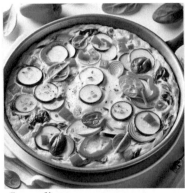

Nutritional Values per Serving:
- Calories: about 180 kcal
- Protein: 18 g
- Fat: 8 g (saturated <2 g)
- Carbohydrates: 5 g
- Fiber: 1 g
- Sugars: 3 g
- Sodium: 300 mg (depends on the amount of salt added)

Preparation Time: 10 minutes
Cooking Time: 10 minutes
Portions: 1

Ingredients:
- Egg whites: 4 large (120 ml or about ½ cup)
- Zucchini: ½ small, diced (about 50 g or 1.75 oz)
- Red peppers: ¼ bell pepper, diced (about 30 g or 1 oz)
- Red onion: ¼ small, chopped (about 25 g or 0.88 oz)
- Fresh spinach: a handful (about 30 g or 1 oz)
- Extra virgin olive oil: 1 teaspoon (5 ml or 1 teaspoon)

Instructions:
Preparing Vegetables:
- Heat olive oil in a nonstick skillet over medium heat.
- Add chopped onion and sauté until translucent, about 2 minutes.
- Add peppers and zucchini, cooking for another 3-4 minutes until softened.
- Add spinach and cook until wilted, about 1 minute.

Frittata Cooking:
- In a bowl, beat egg whites with salt and pepper.
- Pour the beaten egg whites over the vegetables in the pan.
- Cook over medium-low heat, allowing the egg whites to set on the bottom, then shake the pan gently to prevent sticking.
- When the egg whites are almost completely set, but still slightly liquid on the surface, fold the omelet in half or leave it flat, depending on preference.

Finish:
- Continue cooking for another 1 to 2 minutes, until the omelet is completely set.

Tips:
- For a richer version, you can add fresh herbs such as basil or parsley before cooking the egg whites.
- This frittata can be customized with any available seasonal vegetables.

Green detox smoothie

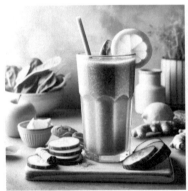

Nutritional Values per Serving:
- Calories: about 140 kcal
- Protein: 2 g
- Fats: 0.5 g
- Carbohydrates: 33 g
- Fiber: 5 g
- Sugars: 25 g
- Sodium: 60 mg

Preparation Time: 10 minutes
Portions: 1

Ingredients:
- Green apple: 1 medium, cut into pieces (about 180 g or 6.3 oz)
- Cucumber: ½ medium, cut into pieces (about 100 g or 3.5 oz)
- Fresh spinach: 1 cup well-pressed (about 30 g or 1 oz)
- Celery: 1 stalk, cut into pieces (about 40 g or 1.4 oz)
- Lemon juice: the juice of ½ lemon (about 2 tablespoons or 30 ml)
- Coconut water: ½ cup (120 ml or 4 oz)
- Fresh ginger: 1 piece of about 2 cm (about 10 g or 0.35 oz)
- Ice cubes: to taste
- If you prefer a more liquid smoothie, add more coconut water to taste.

Instructions:
Preparation:
- Wash all fresh ingredients thoroughly under running water.
- Peel the green apple and remove the core. Cut into small pieces.
- Cut the cucumber and celery into small pieces.
- Peel the ginger and cut it into thin slices.

Blending:
- Put all the ingredients in the blender, adding the coconut water and ice cubes last.
- Blend on high speed until smooth and creamy.

Service:
- Pour the smoothie into a tall glass.
- If you wish, you can garnish with a slice of lemon or a fresh mint leaf for an extra touch of freshness.

Tips:
- For an extra touch of sweetness, you can add a small amount of honey or maple syrup.
- If you prefer a more liquid smoothie, add more coconut water to taste.

Oatmeal and berry porridge

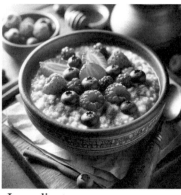

Nutritional Values per Serving:
- Calories: about 250 kcal
- Protein: 6 g
- Fat: 3 g (if you use water; fat content increases if you use milk)
- Carbohydrates: 51 g
- Fiber: 7 g
- Sugars: 15 g (natural from fruits and honey, if any)

Preparation Time: 5 minutes
Cooking Time: 15 minutes
Portions: 1

Ingredients:
- Oatmeal: 1/2 cup (50 g or 1.75 oz)
- Water or milk (for a creamier version): 1 cup (240 ml or 8 oz)
- Mixed berries (raspberries, blueberries, strawberries): ½ cup (about 70 g or 2.5 oz)
- Honey or maple syrup (optional): 1 teaspoon (5 ml or 1 teaspoon)
- A pinch of cinnamon powder

Instructions:
Cooking Oats:
- In a small pot, bring water or milk to a boil.
- Add the oatmeal and reduce the heat.
- Cook, stirring frequently, for about 5 to 10 minutes, until the oats are soft and have absorbed most of the liquid.

Adding the Berries:
- When the oats are almost ready, add the berries to the oatmeal.
- Continue cooking for another 2 to 3 minutes, until the fruits begin to release their juices but are still partly intact.

Service:
- Transfer the porridge to a bowl.
- Add a teaspoon of honey or maple syrup if you want a little more sweetness.
- Sprinkle with a pinch of cinnamon for a touch of spice.

Advice:
- For a gluten-free version, make sure the oats are certified gluten-free.
- You can enrich the oatmeal with chia seeds or flax seeds to add omega-3 and additional fiber.

Tofu scramble with spinach and cherry tomatoes

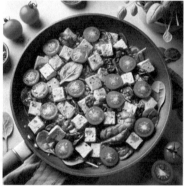

Nutritional Values per Serving:
- Calories: about 250 kcal
- Protein: 18 g
- Fats: 15 g
- Carbohydrates: 10 g
- Fiber: 3 g
- Sugars: 4 g
- Sodium: 200 mg

Preparation Time: 10 minutes
Cooking Time: 12-15 minutes
Portions: 1-2

Ingredients:
- Soft or semi-firm tofu: 200 g (about 7 oz)
- Fresh spinach: 1 cup (about 30 g or 1 oz)
- Tomatoes: ½ cup, cut in half (about 75 g or 2.6 oz)
- Extra virgin olive oil: 1 tablespoon (15 ml or 1 tablespoon)
- Turmeric powder: ½ teaspoon (2 ml or ½ teaspoon) for color
- Salt and ground black pepper: to taste
- Fresh herbs (optional, e.g., basil or parsley): for garnish

Instructions:
Tofu preparation:
- Drain the tofu and pat dry with kitchen paper.
- Crumble it with your hands or a fork into coarse pieces.

Cooking:
- Heat oil in a frying pan over medium heat.
- Add the crumbled tofu and turmeric, mix well to even out the color.
- Cook for about 5 to 7 minutes, until the tofu starts to brown slightly.

Addition of Vegetables:
- Add the spinach and cherry tomatoes to the skillet.
- Cook for another 3 to 5 minutes, until the spinach has wilted and the cherry tomatoes have softened slightly.

Seasoning and Service:
- Season with salt and pepper to taste.
- Serve hot, garnished with fresh herbs if desired.

Tips:
- For a spicy touch, add a pinch of chili powder or a few drops of hot sauce.
- This dish pairs well with whole wheat toast or as a filling for a wrap.

Buckwheat and banana pancakes

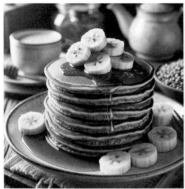

Nutritional Values per Serving:
- Calories: about 300 kcal
- Protein: 8 g
- Fats: 14 g
- Carbohydrates: 38 g
- Fiber: 5 g
- Sugars: 12 g

Preparation Time: 15 minutes
Cooking Time: 6 minutes per batch
Portions: 2-3

Ingredients:
- Buckwheat flour: 1 cup (120 g or 4.2 oz)
- Almond milk (or any milk of your choice): 1 cup (240 ml or 8 oz)
- Ripe banana: 1 large, mashed
- Egg: 1 large
- Coconut oil: 2 tablespoons (30 ml or 2 tablespoons), plus extra for cooking
- Coconut sugar (optional): 1 tablespoon (15 g or 1 tablespoon)
- Baking powder: 1 teaspoon (5 ml or 1 teaspoon)
- Salt: a pinch

Instructions:
Dough Preparation:
- In a large bowl, mix buckwheat flour, baking powder, and salt.
- In another bowl, whisk together the egg, almond milk, coconut oil and mashed banana until smooth.
- Pour the liquid ingredients into the dry ingredients and mix until combined. If the mixture is too thick, add a little more milk.

Pancake baking:
- Heat a nonstick skillet over medium heat and lightly grease with coconut oil.
- Pour about ¼ cup (60 ml) of batter per pancake into the hot pan.
- Cook for 2-3 minutes per side, or until golden brown and bubbles form on the surface before turning them over.

Service:
- Serve the pancakes hot, stacked.
- Garnish with fresh banana slices, a drizzle of maple syrup or honey, and a sprinkle of cinnamon if desired.

Advice:
- For a completely vegan version, replace the egg with ¼ cup applesauce or a vegan egg substitute.
- Add fresh berries to the mix for an extra touch of freshness and flavor.

Chia pudding with coconut milk and mangoes

Nutritional Values per Serving:
- Calories: about 300 kcal
- Protein: 5 g
- Fat: 18 g (dependent on the type of coconut milk used)
- Carbohydrates: 35 g
- Fiber: 8 g
- Sugars: 20 g

Preparation Time: 15 minutes (plus resting time)
Cooking Time: None
Portions: 2

Ingredients:
- Chia seeds: ¼ cup (40 g or 1.4 oz)
- Coconut milk: 1 cup (240 ml or 8 oz)
- Ripe mango: 1 medium, diced (about 200 g or 7 oz)
- Honey or maple syrup (optional): 1 tablespoon (15 ml or 1 tablespoon)
- Vanilla extract: ½ teaspoon (2.5 ml or ½ teaspoon)

Instructions:
Pudding preparation:
- In a medium bowl, combine chia seeds with coconut milk, honey (or maple syrup), and vanilla extract.
- Mix well until everything is well blended.
- Let the mixture sit for at least 4 hours in the refrigerator, preferably overnight, to allow the chia seeds to swell and absorb the liquid, creating a pudding-like consistency.

Mango preparation:
- While the pudding cools, cut the mango into cubes.
- You can choose to leave the mango cubes au naturel or blend them to a puree, depending on your desired consistency.

Assembly:
- Once the pudding has reached the desired consistency, remove it from the refrigerator.
- Arrange a layer of pudding in a glass or bowl.
- Add a layer of mango cubes or mango puree on top of the pudding.
- Repeat the layers until the glass or bowl is full.

Tips:
- For a completely vegan version, make sure the sweetener used is vegan.
- Add a pinch of cinnamon or cardamom for an extra touch of spice.

Oatmeal crepes with apple compote

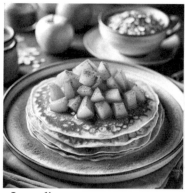

Nutritional Values per Serving:
- Calories: about 350 kcal
- Protein: 9 g
- Fats: 12 g
- Carbohydrates: 53 g
- Fiber: 7 g
- Sugars: 20 g

Preparation Time: 40 minutes (including resting time)
Cooking Time: 30 minutes
Portions: 2-3

Ingredients:
- For the Crepes:
- Oatmeal: 1 cup (90 g or 3.2 oz)
- Almond milk (or any milk of your choice): 1 ½ cups (360 ml-12 oz)
- Large egg: 1
- Melted coconut oil: 1 tablespoon (15 ml or 1 tablespoon), plus extra for cooking
- Vanilla extract: 1 teaspoon (5 ml or 1 teaspoon)
- Salt: a pinch
- For the Apple Compote:
- Large apples, peeled and diced: 2
- Water: ¼ cup (60 ml or 2 oz)
- Cinnamon powder: ½ teaspoon (2.5 ml or ½ teaspoon)
- Clove powder: a pinch
- Lemon juice: 1 tablespoon (15 ml or 1 tablespoon)

Instructions:
Crepes preparation:
- In a blender, combine the oat flour, milk, egg, coconut oil, vanilla extract, and salt. Blend until smooth and homogeneous.
- Let the dough rest for about 20 minutes in the refrigerator to allow the flour to absorb the liquids and thicken slightly.

Cooking Crepes:
- Heat a nonstick skillet over medium heat and grease it lightly with coconut oil.
- Pour about ¼ cup (60 ml) of batter per crepe and tilt the pan to distribute evenly.
- Cook for about 2 minutes per side or until golden brown and easy to turn.

Preparation of Apple Compote:
- In a small pot, combine the apples, water, cinnamon, cloves and lemon juice.
- Cook over medium-low heat, covered, for about 15 to 20 minutes, stirring occasionally, until the apples are soft and most of the liquid has evaporated.

Service:
- Serve the crepes warm, stuffed with the apple compote.
- Optional: add a drizzle of honey or maple syrup for extra sweetness.

Blueberry and dark chocolate chip muffins

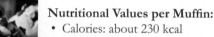

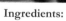

Nutritional Values per Muffin:
- Calories: about 230 kcal
- Protein: 4 g
- Fats: 10 g
- Carbohydrates: 32 g
- Fiber: 2 g
- Sugars: 18 g

Preparation Time: 15 minutes
Baking Time: 25 minutes
Portions: 12 muffins

Ingredients:
- Whole wheat flour: 1 ¾ cups (220 g or 7.8 oz)
- Brown sugar: ¾ cup (150 g or 5.3 oz)
- Yeast powder: 1 teaspoon (5 ml or 1 teaspoon)
- Baking soda: ½ teaspoon (2.5 ml or ½ teaspoon)
- Salt: ½ teaspoon (2.5 ml or ½ teaspoon)
- Eggs: 2 large
- Melted coconut oil: ½ cup (120 ml or 4 oz)
- Greek yogurt: 1 cup (240 ml or 8 oz)
- Vanilla extract: 1 teaspoon (5 ml or 1 teaspoon)
- Fresh blueberries: 1 cup (150 g or 5.3 oz)
- Dark chocolate chips: ½ cup (90 g or 3.2 oz)

Instructions:
Preparation:
- Preheat the oven to 350°F (180°C).
- Line a muffin pan with paper cups or grease it lightly.

Dry Blend:
- In a large bowl, sift together flour, brown sugar, baking powder, baking soda, and salt.

Wet Blend:
- In another bowl, beat the eggs with the coconut oil, Greek yogurt and vanilla extract until smooth.

Combination of Ingredients:
- Add the wet mixture to the dry mixture and mix until the ingredients are just combined.
- Gently, incorporate the blueberries and chocolate chips.

Cooking:
- Spread the batter into the ramekins, filling them up to ¾ full.
- Bake for 20 to 25 minutes or until a toothpick inserted in the center of a muffin comes out clean.

Cooling:
- Let the muffins cool in the pan for 5 minutes, then transfer them to a wire rack to complete cooling.

Tips:
- Be sure not to over-mix the batter to keep the muffins soft and fluffy.
- You can substitute blueberries and chocolate for other fruits or types of chocolate depending on your preference.

Egg White Omelet

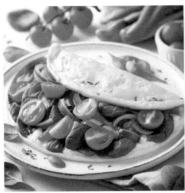

Nutritional Values per Serving:
- Calories: about 150 kcal
- Protein: 15 g
- Fats: 5 g
- Carbohydrates: 5 g
- Fiber: 1 g
- Sugars: 2 g

Preparation Time: 10 minutes
Cooking Time: 10 minutes
Portions: 1

Ingredients:
- Egg whites: 4 large
- Fresh spinach: ½ cup (about 15 g or 0.5 oz)
- Tomatoes: ½ cup, cut in half (about 75 g or 2.6 oz)
- Red onion: ¼, thinly sliced (about 25 g or 0.88 oz)
- Peppers: ¼ bell pepper, cut into strips (about 30 g or 1 oz)
- Olive oil: 1 teaspoon (5 ml or 1 teaspoon)
- Salt and pepper: to taste

Instructions:
Preparation of Ingredients:
- Wash and prepare spinach, cherry tomatoes, onion, and peppers as directed.

Cooking Vegetables:
- Heat olive oil in a nonstick skillet over medium heat.
- Add onion and bell bell pepper, cooking until soft and slightly caramelized, about 3-4 minutes.
- Add spinach and cherry tomatoes, cook until spinach wilts, about 1-2 minutes.

Cooking the Omelette:
- In a bowl, lightly beat the egg whites with salt and pepper.
- Pour the egg whites over the pan with the already cooked vegetables.
- Cook over medium-low heat without stirring, allowing the omelet to set on the bottom and sides, about 2-3 minutes.
- Using a spatula, gently lift the edges of the omelet and tilt the pan to drain the uncapped liquid to the bottom.

Service:
- Once the omelet is completely set but still moist on the surface, fold it in half.
- Serve immediately.

Tips:
- Customize the omelet by adding fresh herbs or spices such as curry to vary the flavor.
- For a more substantial meal, accompany the omelet with a slice of toasted whole wheat bread.

Matcha tea and kiwi smoothie bowl

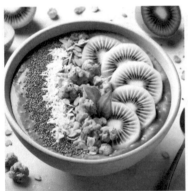

Nutritional Values per Serving:
- Calories: about 350 kcal
- Protein: 5 g
- Fats: 14 g
- Carbohydrates: 55 g
- Fiber: 8 g
- Sugars: 35 g

Preparation Time: 10 minutes
Portions: 1-2

Ingredients:
- Coconut milk: 1 cup (240 ml or 8 oz)
- Matcha tea powder: 1 teaspoon (5 ml or 1 teaspoon)
- Ripe banana: 1, frozen
- Kiwis: 2, peeled and cut into pieces
- Honey: 1 tablespoon (15 ml or 1 tablespoon)
- Ice: ½ cup (about 120 ml or 4 oz)

To garnish:
- Kiwi slices
- Crunchy granola
- Chia seeds
- Cocchi flakes

Instructions:
Preparing the Smoothie:
- In a blender, combine coconut milk, matcha tea powder, frozen banana, one kiwi, honey and ice.
- Blend until smooth and creamy. If necessary, add a little more milk to achieve the desired consistency.

Assembling the Smoothie Bowl:
- Pour the smoothie into a large bowl.
- Garnish with kiwi slices, crunchy granola, chia seeds and coconut flakes.

Service:
- Serve immediately to enjoy the freshness and creaminess of the smoothie bowl.

Tips:
- For a touch of additional protein, consider adding a scoop of protein powder to the shake.
- Vary fruit and toppings to diversify flavors and nutrients.

Greek yogurt with nuts and berries

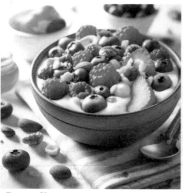

Nutritional Values per Serving:
- Calories: about 350 kcal
- Protein: 20 g
- Fats: 18 g
- Carbohydrates: 25 g
- Fiber: 3 g
- Sugars: 18 g

Preparation Time: 10 minutes
Portions: 1

Ingredients:
- Greek yogurt: 1 cup (about 245 g or 8.6 oz)
- Mixed fresh berries (blueberries, raspberries, strawberries): ½ cup (about 70 g or 2.5 oz)
- Mixed nuts, lightly roasted (walnuts, almonds, pecans): ¼ cup (about 30 g or 1 oz)
- Honey: 1 tablespoon (15 ml or 1 tablespoon) (optional)

Instructions:
Preparation:
- If not already ready, lightly toast walnuts in a skillet over medium-low heat for 3 to 5 minutes, until lightly browned and aromatic. Let them cool and then coarsely chop them.

Assembly:
- In a bowl, pour the Greek yogurt.
- Add washed and dried berries on top of the yogurt.
- Sprinkle the toasted walnuts on top of the berries.
- Drizzle it with honey if you want some additional sweetness.

Service:
- Serve immediately to enjoy the freshness of the fruit and the crunchiness of the nuts.

Tips:
- For a vegan version, substitute Greek yogurt for a coconut or almond-based yogurt.
- Vary the berries according to the season to keep the dish fresh and interesting

Avocado toast with poached egg and cherry tomatoes

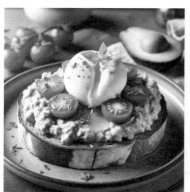

Nutritional Values per Serving:
- Calories: about 400 kcal
- Protein: 15 g
- Fats: 30 g
- Carbohydrates: 27 g
- Fiber: 9 g
- Sugars: 4 g

Preparation Time: 20 minutes
Cooking Time: 10 minutes
Portions: 2

Ingredients:
- Slices of whole wheat bread: 2
- Ripe avocado: 1 large
- Eggs: 2
- Tomatoes: 1 cup, cut in half (about 150 g or 5.3 oz)
- Extra virgin olive oil: for garnish
- Salt and ground black pepper: to taste
- Lemon juice: 1 teaspoon (5 ml or 1 teaspoon)
- Fresh herbs (basil or parsley): for garnish

Instructions:
Bread preparation:
- Toast the bread slices until they are crisp and golden brown.

Avocado Preparation:
- Cut the avocado in half, remove the pit, and scoop out the pulp with a spoon.
- In a bowl, mash the avocado with a fork until creamy.
- Season with salt, pepper and a little lemon juice.

Cooking the Poached Egg:
- Bring a pot of water with a pinch of salt to a boil.
- Reduce to a gentle simmer and add a tablespoon of vinegar (helps coagulate the egg white).
- Gently crack the egg into a cup, then slide the egg into the water.
- Let cook for 3-4 minutes for a still-liquid yolk.
- Use a skimmer to remove the egg from the water and let it drain on kitchen paper.

Assembly:
- Spread the mashed avocado on the toasted bread slices.
- Gently lay a poached egg on each slice.
- Add the chopped cherry tomatoes on top of the egg.
- Garnish with a drizzle of olive oil, salt, pepper and fresh herbs.

Tips:
- For a spicy touch, add a sprinkling of chili powder or a few drops of hot sauce.
- Experiment with different types of bread, such as rye or multigrain, for variations on the theme.

Overnight oats with peanut butter and banana

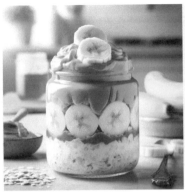

Nutritional Values per Serving:
- Calories: about 450 kcal
- Protein: 15 g
- Fat: 18 g (dependent on the type of peanut butter used)
- Carbohydrates: 60 g
- Fiber: 8 g
- Sugars: 20 g

Preparation Time: 10 minutes
Refrigeration Time: 6 hours or more
Portions: 1

Ingredients:
- Oatmeal: 1/2 cup (50 g or 1.75 oz)
- Almond milk (or other milk of choice): ½ cup (120 ml or 4 oz)
- Greek yogurt: ¼ cup (60 ml or 2 oz)
- Peanut butter: 2 tablespoons (30 ml or 2 tablespoons)
- Ripe banana: 1, mashed
- Honey (optional): 1 tablespoon (15 ml or 1 tablespoon)
- Chia seeds: 1 teaspoon (5 ml or 1 teaspoon)

Instructions:
Preparation:
- In a jar or bowl, combine oatmeal, almond milk, Greek yogurt, peanut butter, mashed banana, honey, and chia seeds.
- Mix well until all ingredients are fully combined.

Refrigeration:
- Cover the jar or bowl with a lid or plastic wrap.
- Let sit in the refrigerator overnight, or at least for 6 hours, so that the oats can absorb the liquids and soften.

Service:
- In the morning, take the contents out of the refrigerator.
- If the oats appear too thick, you can add a little more milk to reach the desired consistency.
- Mix well before serving.
- Add additional fresh banana slices or another tablespoon of peanut butter on top for garnish, if desired.

Tips:
- Experiment by adding other ingredients such as dried fruits, other seeds or spices such as cinnamon to vary the flavors.
- For a completely vegan version, make sure the yogurt and honey are suitable for vegans or replace them with vegan alternatives.

Oatmeal and berry tart

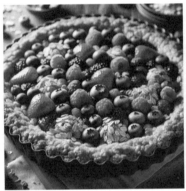

Nutritional Values per Serving:
- Calories: about 280 kcal
- Protein: 4 g
- Fats: 12 g
- Carbohydrates: 42 g
- Fiber: 4 g
- Sugars: 22 g

Preparation Time: 20 minutes
Cooking Time: 45 minutes
Portions: 8

Ingredients:
- For the base:
- Oatmeal: 1 cup (90 g or 3.2 oz)
- Whole wheat flour: ½ cup (60 g or 2.1 oz)
- Cold butter, cubed: ½ cup (115 g or 4 oz)
- Brown sugar: ¼ cup (50 g or 1.76 oz)
- Salt: a pinch
- For the filling:
- Mixed berries (blueberries, raspberries, cut strawberries): 2 cups (about 300 g or 10.6 oz)
- Brown sugar: ½ cup (100 g or 3.5 oz)
- Cornstarch: 1 tablespoon (8 g or 0.28 oz)
- Lemon juice: 1 tablespoon (15 ml or 1 tablespoon)

Instructions:
Preparation of the Base:
- Preheat the oven to 350°F (180°C).
- In a bowl, mix oatmeal, flour, brown sugar and salt.
- Add the butter and process the mixture with your hands or a mixer until it has a sandy consistency.
- Press the mixture into a tart pan, forming a high rim on the sides.

Preparing the Stuffing:
- In a bowl, combine the berries with the brown sugar, cornstarch and lemon juice.
- Mix gently until everything is well combined.
- Pour the filling over the oat base in the baking dish.

Cooking:
- Bake for about 40-45 minutes or until the filling is hot and the base is golden brown.
- Let cool completely before serving to allow the filling to thicken.

Tips:
- For an even healthier variation, replace the butter with coconut oil and reduce the amount of sugar in the filling.
- You can use any combination of fresh or frozen berries, depending on availability and preference.
-

Savory quinoa and zucchini pancakes

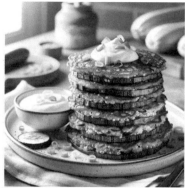

Nutritional Values per Serving:
- Calories: about 250 kcal
- Protein: 10 g
- Fats: 10 g
- Carbohydrates: 30 g
- Fiber: 4 g
- Sugars: 3 g

Preparation Time: 20 minutes
Cooking Time: 8 minutes per batch
Portions: 4

Ingredients:
- Cooked quinoa: 1 cup (about 185 g or 6.5 oz)
- Large zucchini: 1, grated (about 200 g or 7 oz)
- Whole wheat flour: ½ cup (60 g or 2.1 oz)
- Eggs: 2 large
- Grated Parmesan cheese: ¼ cup (about 30 g or 1 oz)
- Green onion: 2, finely chopped
- Garlic: 1 clove, chopped
- Salt and black pepper: to taste
- Olive oil: for cooking

Instructions:
Preparation of Mixture:
- In a large bowl, mix cooked quinoa, grated zucchini, whole wheat flour, eggs, Parmesan cheese, green onions, garlic, salt, and pepper until smooth.

Pancake Baking:
- Heat a drizzle of olive oil in a nonstick skillet over medium heat.
- Pour about ¼ cup (60 ml) of the mixture for each pancake into the hot pan.
- Cook for 3-4 minutes per side, until golden brown and well cooked.

Service:
- Serve the pancakes hot, accompanied by Greek yogurt or a sauce of your choice to add a cool touch.

Tips:
- Be sure to squeeze the grated zucchini well to remove excess water before adding them to the mixture to avoid pancakes that are too wet.
- Vary the ingredients by adding other vegetables such as carrots or spinach to diversify the taste and nutrients

Lemon Ricotta Pancakes

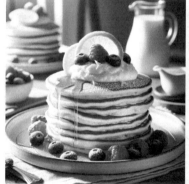

Nutritional Information per Serving:
- Calories: approximately 250 kcal
- Protein: 12 g
- Fat: 10 g
- Carbohydrates: 28 g
- Fiber: 4 g
- Sugars: 8 g

Preparation Time: 10 minutes
Cooking Time: 15 minutes
Servings: 4

Ingredients:
- Oat flour: 100 g (3.5 oz)
- Ricotta cheese: 150 g (5.3 oz)
- Milk: 120 ml (4 fl oz / 0.5 cup)
- Eggs: 2
- Lemon zest: 1 tablespoon (from one lemon)
- Lemon juice: 1 tablespoon
- Baking powder: 1 teaspoon
- Honey: 2 tablespoons (optional)
- Extra virgin olive oil: for cooking
- Berries: for serving
- Maple syrup: for serving

Instructions:
- Prepare the Batter:
- In a large bowl, mix the oat flour, ricotta cheese, milk, eggs, lemon zest, lemon juice, and baking powder until well combined. If you prefer a sweeter batter, add the honey.
-
- Cook the Pancakes:
- Heat a non-stick skillet over medium heat and add a drizzle of extra virgin olive oil.
- Pour a ladleful of batter into the hot skillet and cook for 2-3 minutes, until the edges start to set and bubbles form on the surface.
- Flip the pancake and cook the other side for another 2-3 minutes, until golden brown.
- Repeat the process with the remaining batter.

Serve:
- Serve the pancakes warm with fresh berries and a drizzle of maple syrup.

Tips:
- For a gluten-free option, use certified gluten-free oat flour.
- Add chia seeds or flaxseeds to the batter for extra fiber and omega-3s.

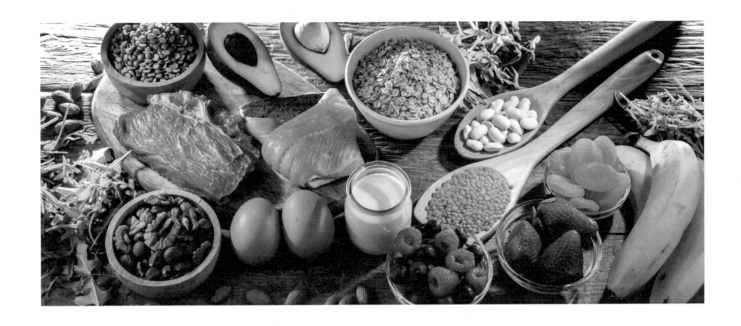

CHAPTER 8: LIGHT AND NUTRITIOUS LUNCHES

8.1 Criteria for choosing lunches suitable for fatty liver

When selecting main meals for those suffering from fatty liver, it is crucial to consider a few critical criteria. The goal is to provide the body with essential nutrients while maintaining a balanced caloric intake and promoting liver health. Here are the main criteria to consider:

1. Lean protein: Opt for lean protein sources such as chicken, turkey, fish, legumes, tofu, and eggs. Limit consumption of red and processed meats, which can increase inflammation and workload for the liver.
2. Healthy fats: Include sources of healthy fats such as avocados, nuts, seeds, olive oil, and fatty fish (salmon, mackerel, sardines). These fats provide essential fatty acids and support liver health, but should be consumed in moderation.
3. Complex carbohydrates: Choose carbohydrates such as brown rice, quinoa, spelled, sweet potatoes, and legumes. These foods provide sustained energy, fiber, and essential nutrients while avoiding glycemic spikes that can stress the liver.
4. Abundance of vegetables: Include a variety of non-starchy vegetables in every meal. Vegetables are rich in fiber, vitamins, minerals, and antioxidants that support liver function and promote detoxification.
5. Controlled portions: Pay attention to portion size to avoid excessive caloric intake. Use smaller plates and divide servings evenly between protein, complex carbohydrates, and vegetables.
6. Limit sugars and saturated fats: Minimize consumption of added sugars, sweets, sugary drinks, and processed foods high in saturated fats. These foods can contribute to fat accumulation and inflammation in the liver.
7. Herbs and spices: Use a variety of herbs and spices to flavor dishes, such as turmeric, ginger, garlic, coriander, and rosemary. These ingredients have antioxidant and anti-inflammatory properties that can support liver health.
8. Healthy cooking methods: Opt for healthy cooking methods such as steaming, baking, grilling, or quick sautéing. Avoid frying or prolonged cooking at high temperatures, which can generate liver-damaging substances.
9. Adequate hydration: Drink enough water throughout the day to support liver function and promote the elimination of toxins. Avoid alcoholic beverages, which can damage the liver.
10. Regular meals: Maintain a regular meal routine, avoiding skipping or binge eating. This helps keep blood sugar levels stable and reduces stress on the liver.

Following these criteria when choosing lunches makes balanced and tasty meals that support liver health and promote the body's overall well-being possible. In the following sections, we will explore specific recipes embodying these principles.

Quinoa Salad with Tuna, Avocado and Tomatoes

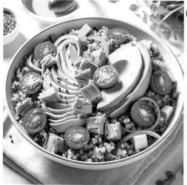

Nutritional Values per Serving:
- Calories: about 400 kcal
- Protein: 22 g
- Fat: 22 g (dependent on the type of oil and fat content of the avocado)
- Carbohydrates: 35 g
- Fiber: 8 g
- Sugars: 5 g

**Preparation Time: 25 minutes
(plus cooling time for quinoa)
Portions: 2-3**

Ingredients:
- Quinoa: 1 cup (about 170 g or 6 oz), cooked
- Natural canned tuna: 1 can (about 140 g or 5 oz),
- Avocado: 1, ripe, diced
- Cherry tomatoes: 1 cup (about 150 g or 5.3 oz), cut in half.
- Red onion: ¼ small, thinly sliced.
- Lemon juice: 2 tablespoons (30 ml or 2 tablespoons)
- Extra virgin olive oil: 2 tablespoons (30 ml or 2 tablespoons)
- Salt and ground black pepper: to taste
- Fresh herbs (such as parsley or cilantro): chopped, for garnish.

Instructions:
Preparation of Quinoa:
- If not already cooked, rinse quinoa well under running water, then cook it in boiling salted water following the instructions on the package, usually about 15 minutes. Let it cool completely.

Composition of the Salad:
- In a large bowl, mix cooled quinoa, drained tuna, diced avocado, chopped cherry tomatoes, and sliced red onion.
- In a small bowl, emulsify lemon juice with olive oil, salt and pepper.
- Pour the dressing over the salad and toss gently to combine all the ingredients.

Service:
- Garnish the salad with chopped fresh herbs before serving.
- It can be served immediately or stored in the refrigerator for a few hours to intensify the flavors.

Tips:
- For a vegetarian variation, replace the tuna with chickpeas or another legume to maintain the protein content.
- Add a touch of spice with some chopped fresh chili or dried chili flakes.

Lettuce Wrap with Grilled Salmon, Cucumbers and Yogurt Sauce

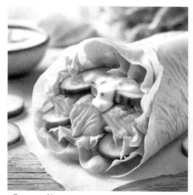

Nutritional Values per Serving:
- Calories: about 300 kcal
- Protein: 23 g
- Fat: 15 g (dependent on the type of yogurt and the amount of oil used)
- Carbohydrates: 8 g
- Fiber: 2 g
- Sugars: 4 g

**Preparation Time: 20 minutes
Cooking Time: 8 minutes
Portions: 2-3**

Ingredients:
- Salmon: 2 fillets (about 200 g or 7 oz each)
- Romaine or iceberg lettuce: 6-8 large leaves, washed and dried
- Cucumbers: 1 medium, cut into strips
- Greek yogurt: ½ cup (120 ml or 4 oz)
- Lemon: the juice of 1 lemon
- Garlic: 1 clove, finely chopped
- Fresh dill: 1 tablespoon chopped
- Salt and pepper: to taste
- Olive oil: for grilling

For the Yogurt Sauce:
- Mix Greek yogurt, lemon juice, minced garlic, dill, salt and pepper in a bowl until smooth.

Instructions:
Preparation of Salmon:
- Preheat the grill to medium-high temperature.
- Season the salmon fillets with salt, pepper and a drizzle of olive oil.
- Grill the salmon for about 3-4 minutes per side, or until it is well cooked and flakes easily with a fork.
- Once cooked, let it cool slightly and shred it with a fork.

Wrap assembly:
- Extend the lettuce leaves on a plate.
- Spread the shredded grilled salmon in the center of each leaf.
- Add the cucumber strips on top of the salmon.
- Pour a spoonful of yogurt sauce over each wrap.

Service:
- Roll up the lettuce leaves to close the wrap. Serve immediately to enjoy the freshness of the ingredients.

Tips:
- For a spicier variation, add fresh chopped chili peppers or a pinch of cayenne pepper to the yogurt sauce wrap.
- Experiment with different fresh herbs in the sauce, such as cilantro or parsley, to vary the flavors.

Lentil and Vegetable Soup in a Carrier Cup

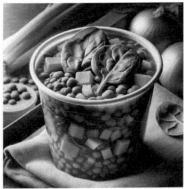

Nutritional Values per Serving:
- Calories: about 250 kcal
- Protein: 12 g
- Fats: 5 g
- Carbohydrates: 40 g
- Fiber: 10 g
- Sugars: 8 g

Preparation Time: 15 minutes
Cooking Time: 35 minutes
Portions: 4

Ingredients:
- Lentils: 1 cup (200 g or 7 oz), rinsed and drained
- Carrots: 2 medium, peeled and diced
- Celery: 2 stalks, cut into pieces
- Onion: 1 medium, chopped
- Garlic: 2 cloves, chopped
- Canned peeled tomatoes: 1 can (400 g or 14 oz)
- Vegetable broth: 4 cups (1 L)
- Extra virgin olive oil: 2 tablespoons (30 ml)
- Salt and black pepper: to taste
- Rosemary: 1 sprig
- Thyme: 1 sprig
- Fresh spinach: 1 cup (30 g or 1 oz)

Instructions:
Soup Preparation:
- In a large pot, heat olive oil over medium heat. Add the onion, carrot, celery, and garlic, and sauté until soft, about 5 minutes.
- Add the lentils, peeled tomatoes, vegetable stock, rosemary, and thyme. Bring to a boil, then reduce heat and simmer for about 30 minutes, or until lentils are tender.
- Add spinach in the last few minutes of cooking, letting it wilt in the soup.

Service:
- Remove the rosemary and thyme before serving.
- Taste and adjust salt and pepper as needed.
- Pour the soup into thermal take-out cups to keep the heat in.

Advice:
- For a spicier version, add a sprinkling of smoked paprika or chili powder while cooking.
- You can add other vegetables as desired, such as zucchini or bell peppers, to further enrich the nutritional content of the soup.

Shrimp Tacos with Avocado Salsa and Coleslaw

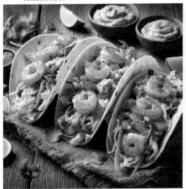

Nutritional Values per Serving:
- Calories: about 350 kcal
- Protein: 25 g
- Fats: 15 g
- Carbohydrates: 35 g
- Fiber: 6 g
- Sugars: 5 g

Preparation Time: 30 minutes
Cooking Time: 10 minutes
Portions: 4

Tips:
- For a spicy touch, add crushed chili to the avocado sauce or a pinch of cayenne pepper to the shrimp before cooking them.

Ingredients:
- For the Prawns:
- Fresh or frozen shrimp, shelled and cleaned: 400 g (about 14 oz)
- Olive oil: 1 tablespoon (15 ml)
- Smoked paprika: 1 teaspoon (5 ml)
- Garlic powder: 1 teaspoon (5 ml)
- Salt and pepper: to taste
- For the Avocado Sauce:
- Ripe avocado: 1 large
- Lime juice: from 1 lime
- Chopped fresh coriander: 1 handful
- Salt and pepper: to taste

For the Coleslaw:
- Green cabbage, finely chopped: 2 cups (about 150 g or 5 oz)
- Carrots, grated: ½ cup (about 50 g or 1.75 oz)
- Extra virgin olive oil: 2 tablespoons (30 ml
- Apple vinegar: 1 tablespoon (15 ml)
- Honey: 1 tspin
- Salt and pepper: to taste
- To Assemble:
- Corn tortillas: 8 small

Instructions:
Preparation of Shrimp:
- In a bowl, mix shrimp with olive oil, paprika, garlic powder, salt and pepper.
- Heat a skillet over medium-high heat and cook the shrimp for 2-3 minutes per side, until they are pink and cooked through.

Preparation of Avocado Sauce:
- Mash the avocado in a bowl and mix with the lime juice, chopped cilantro, salt and pepper until creamy.

Preparation of Kale Salad:
- In a large bowl, mix the cabbage and carrots.
- In a small bowl, combine olive oil, apple cider vinegar, honey, salt and pepper to make the dressing.
- Pour the dressing over the coleslaw and mix well.

Assembly of Tacos:
- Heat the tortillas in a frying pan or in the microwave.
- Spread the coleslaw over the warm tortillas.
- Add the cooked shrimp.
- Top with a spoonful of avocado salsa on each taco.

Wholewheat Pasta Salad with Chicken, Pesto and Peas.

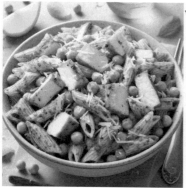

- Nutritional Values per Serving:
- Calories: about 450 kcal
- Protein: 28 g
- Fats: 15 g
- Carbohydrates: 50 g
- Fiber: 6 g
- Sugars: 3 g

Preparation Time: 20 minutes
Cooking Time: 15 minutes
Portions: 4

Ingredients:
- Whole wheat pasta (penne or fusilli): 250 g (about 8.8 oz)
- Chicken breast: 2 medium, cooked and diced
- Pesto: ¼ cup (about 60 ml or 2 oz)
- Fresh or frozen peas: 1 cup (about 150 g or 5.3 oz)
- Extra virgin olive oil: 2 tablespoons (30 ml)
- Grated Parmesan cheese: 2 tablespoons (about 30 g or 1 oz)
- Salt and pepper: to taste
- Lemon: i

Instructions:
Cooking Pasta:
- Bring a large pot of salted water to a boil.
- Cook whole wheat pasta according to the instructions on the package until al dente.
- If you use fresh peas, add them to the pasta cooking water in the last 3 minutes.
- Drain pasta and peas and rinse under cold water to stop cooking.

Preparation of Other Ingredients:
- In a large bowl, mix the cooked chicken, cooled pasta, peas, pesto, Parmesan, lemon juice, and olive oil.
- Season with salt and pepper to taste.

Service:
- Mix all ingredients well before serving.
- You can serve this salad cold or at room temperature.
- Garnish with additional grated Parmesan cheese or a few leaves of fresh basil if desired.

Tips:
- For a vegetarian version, replace the chicken with chickpeas or another legume to maintain the protein content.
- Vary the vegetables by adding baby spinach or arugula for an extra touch of freshness.

Open sandwich with scrambled eggs, spinach and low-fat cheese

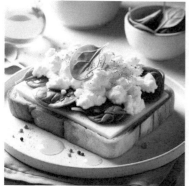

Nutritional Values per Serving:
- Calories: about 350 kcal
- Protein: 25 g
- Fats: 15 g
- Carbohydrates: 30 g
- Fiber: 6 g
- Sugars: 4 g

Preparation Time: 15 minutes
Cooking Time: 10 minutes
Portions: 2

Ingredients:
- Whole wheat bread: 2 slices
- Eggs: 4
- Fresh spinach: 1 cup (about 30 g or 1 oz)
- Low-fat cheese (such as mozzarella or fresh goat cheese): ½ cup grated (about 50 g or 1.75 oz)
- Olive oil: 1 teaspoon (5 ml)
- Salt and black pepper: to taste

Instructions:
Bread preparation:
- Toast slices of whole wheat bread until crisp and golden brown.

Cooking Eggs and Spinach:
- Heat olive oil in a nonstick skillet over medium heat.
- Add spinach and cook until wilted, about 1 to 2 minutes.
- In a bowl, beat the eggs with salt and pepper.
- Pour the eggs into the pan with the spinach and cook, stirring gently, until the eggs are fully cooked but still soft.

Assembly of the Sandwich:
- Arrange the scrambled eggs and spinach on the toasted bread slices.
- Sprinkle grated cheese over the eggs while they are still warm to allow the cheese to melt slightly.

Service:
- Serve the open sandwich immediately, adding an extra pinch of pepper if desired.

Advice:
- For a richer variation, add sun-dried tomatoes or sliced avocado on top of the eggs before adding the cheese.
- Experiment with different types of bread, such as cereal or spelt bread, for variations on the theme.

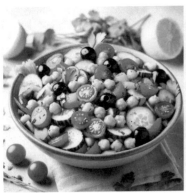

Chickpea Salad with Mixed Vegetables and Lemon Vinaigrette

Nutritional Values per Serving:
- Calories: about 280 kcal
- Protein: 8 g
- Fats: 18 g
- Carbohydrates: 24 g
- Fiber: 6 g
- Sugars: 5 g

Preparation Time: 20 minutes
Portions: 4

Ingredients:
- Chickpeas: 1 can (400 g or 14 oz), rinsed and drained
- Cherry tomatoes: 1 cup (about 150 g or 5.3 oz), cut in half
- Cucumber: 1 medium, diced
- Bell peppers: 1 red, diced
- Red onion: ¼ small, finely sliced
- Black olives: ½ cup (about 70 g or 2.5 oz), pitted and cut in half
- Fresh herbs (such as parsley or cilantro): 3 tablespoons chopped
- Salt and black pepper: to taste

For the Lemon Vinaigrette:
- Extra virgin olive oil: ¼ cup (60 ml)
- Fresh lemon juice: 3 tablespoons (45 ml)
- White wine vinegar: 1 tablespoon (15 ml)
- Dijon mustard: 1 teaspoon (5 ml)
- Garlic: 1 clove, finely chopped
- Salt and pepper: to taste

Instructions:
Preparation of Vinaigrette:

- In a small bowl, combine the olive oil, lemon juice, white wine vinegar, Dijon mustard, minced garlic, salt, and pepper.
- Mix well until a smooth emulsion is obtained.

Salad composition:
- In a large bowl, combine the chickpeas, cherry tomatoes, cucumber, red bell bell pepper, red onion, black olives, and chopped fresh herbs.
- Pour the lemon vinaigrette over the salad and toss gently to combine all the ingredients.

Service:
- Taste and adjust salt and pepper if necessary.
- Let the salad sit for at least 10 minutes before serving to allow the flavors to meld.

Advice:
- For a richer variation, add crumbled feta cheese or diced avocado.
- This salad keeps well in the refrigerator, making it perfect for lunches prepared in advance.

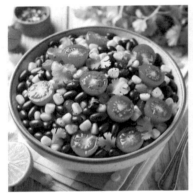

Black Bean Salad with Corn, Tomatoes and Cilantro

Nutritional Values per Serving:
- Calories: about 200 kcal
- Protein: 8 g
- Fat: 7 g
- Carbohydrates: 28 g
- Fiber: 8 g
- Sugars: 5 g

Preparation Time: 15 minutes
Resting Time: 30 minutes
Portions: 4

Ingredients:
- Black beans: 1 can (400 g or 14 oz), rinsed and drained
- Corn: 1 cup (about 175 g or 6 oz), cooked
- Cherry tomatoes: 1 cup (about 150 g or 5.3 oz), cut in half
- Red onion: ¼ small, finely chopped
- Fresh cilantro: ¼ cup (about 4 g or 0.14 oz), chopped
- Jalapeño pepper: 1 small, finely chopped (optional)
- Extra virgin olive oil: 2 tablespoons (30 ml)
- Lime juice: from 2 limes
- Salt and pepper: to taste

Instructions:
1Preparing the Salad:
- In a large bowl, combine the black beans, corn, cherry tomatoes, red onion, chopped cilantro, and jalapeño pepper, if using.

Dressing Preparation:
- In a small bowl, mix olive oil, lime juice, salt, and pepper until emulsified.
- Pour the dressing over the salad and mix well to combine all the ingredients.

Service:
- Let the salad rest in the refrigerator for at least 30 minutes before serving to allow the flavors to meld.
- Taste and adjust salt and pepper, if necessary, before serving.

Advice:
- For a touch of crunch, add toasted pumpkin seeds or sunflower seeds at the time of serving.
- This salad keeps well in the refrigerator, making it perfect for lunches prepared in advance.

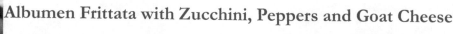

Albumen Frittata with Zucchini, Peppers and Goat Cheese

- Nutritional Values per Serving:
- Calories: about 150 kcal
- Protein: 14 g
- Fat: 9 g (dependent on cheese and oil used)
- Carbohydrates: 3 g
- Fiber: 1 g
- Sugar: 3g

Preparation Time: 15 minutes
Cooking Time: 10 minutes
Portions: 2-3

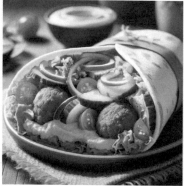

Ingredients:
- Albumens: 6
- Zucchini: 1 small, thinly sliced
- Red bell pepper: 1 small, cut into strips
- Goat cheese: 50 g (about 1.75 oz), crumbled
- Olive oil: 1 tablespoon (15 ml)
- Salt and pepper: to taste
- Fresh herbs (such as basil or thyme): for garnish

Instructions:
Preparing Vegetables:
- Heat olive oil in a nonstick skillet over medium heat.
- Add zucchini and bell pepper, cooking until soft, about 5-7 minutes.

Frittata Cooking:
- In a bowl, beat egg whites with a pinch of salt and pepper.
- Pour the egg whites into the pan with the vegetables.
- Cook over medium-low heat, allowing the egg whites to set on the bottom. Do not stir.
- When the egg whites are almost set but still slightly liquid on top, sprinkle the crumbled goat cheese over the top.

Finish:
- Cover the pan with a lid and cook for another 2 to 3 minutes, until the omelet is completely set and the cheese has begun to melt.
- Garnish with fresh herbs before serving.

Service:
- Serve the omelet hot, cut into wedges.

Tips:
- For a richer omelet, you can add other vegetables such as spinach or mushrooms.
- This recipe is easily adapted to be baked as well, for a version more like a quiche without a crust.

Hummus Wrap with Falafel and Mixed Salad

Nutritional Values per Serving:
- Calories: about 400 kcal
- Protein: 13 g
- Fats: 20 g
- Carbohydrates: 45 g
- Fiber: 6 g
- Sugars: 5 g

Preparation Time: 20 minutes
Portions: 4

Ingredients:
- Flour tortillas: 4
- Hummus: 1 cup (about 240 ml or 8 oz)
- Falafel (already cooked, available at the supermarket or home-made): 12 pieces
- Romaine lettuce: 2 cups, str
- Tomatoes: ½ cup (about 75 g or 2.6 oz), cut in half
- Cucumber: 1 small, thinly sliced
- Red onion: ¼, thinly sliced
- Tahini sauce: ¼ cup (about 60 m

Instructions:
Preparation of Components:
- If the falafel is not already cooked, follow the instructions on the package to cook it until it is crispy on the outside and warm on the inside.

Assembly of Wraps:
- Heat the tortillas in a skillet over medium heat to make them more pliable.
- Spread a generous amount of hummus on each tortilla.
- Spread the hot falafel along the center of each tortilla.
- Add lettuce, cherry tomatoes, cucumber and red onion on top
- Drizzle the tahini sauce over the vegetables.

Closure and Service:
- Roll the tortillas around the filling, folding the edges to close the sides if necessary.
- Cut each wrap in half and serve immediately to enjoy maximum freshness and crispness.
- Tips:
- For a gluten-free variation, use corn or other grain-based gluten-free tortillas.
- Add sliced jalapeño peppers or a little hot sauce if you prefer a spicy touch.

Grilled Chicken Salad with Avocado, Tomatoes and Walnuts

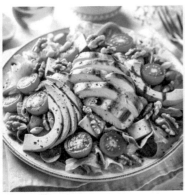

Nutritional Values per Serving:
- Calories: about 350 kcal
- Protein: 25 g
- Fat: 20 g (dependent on oil and nuts)
- Carbohydrates: 15 g
- Fiber: 5 g
- Sugars: 5 g

Preparation Time: 30 minutes
Cooking Time: 15 minutes
Portions: 4

Ingredients:
- Chicken breast: 2 medium (about 400 g or 14 oz)
- Avocado: 1 large, ripe, diced
- Cherry tomatoes: 1 cup (about 150 g or 5.3 oz), cut in half
- Walnuts: ¼ cup (about 30 g or 1 oz), toasted and coarsely chopped
- Green salad mix (such as romaine lettuce, arugula, spinach): 4 cups
- Olive oil: for grilling and seasoning
- Balsamic vinegar: 2 tablespoons (30 ml)
- Lemon juice: 1 tablespoon (15 ml)
- Salt and black pepper: to taste

Instructions:
Preparation of Chicken:
- Season the chicken breasts with salt, pepper and a drizzle of olive oil.
- Grill the chicken on a hot grill or grill pan for about 5 to 7 minutes per side, or until it is well cooked and has a nice golden crust.
- Let the chicken rest for a few minutes, then cut it into strips or cubes.

Salad preparation:
- In a large bowl, combine the green salad mix, diced avocado, cherry tomatoes, and toasted walnuts.
- In a small bowl, mix olive oil, balsamic vinegar, and lemon juice to create the dressing.
- Dress the salad with the dressing and toss gently to combine all the ingredients.

Assembly and Service:
- Arrange the salad on serving plates.
- Add the grilled chicken on top of the salad.
- Season with an additional pinch of salt and pepper, if desired, before serving.

Tips:
- For a richer variation, add feta cheese or parmesan shavings.
- Vary the vegetables according to the season to keep the salad fresh and interesting.

Spelt Salad with Shrimp, Tomatoes and Basil

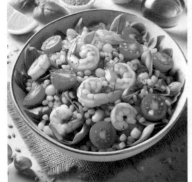

Nutritional Values per Serving:
- Calories: about 350 kcal
- Protein: 25 g
- Fats: 12 g
- Carbohydrates: 35 g
- Fiber: 6 g
- Sugars: 3 g

Preparation Time: 30 minutes
Cooking Time: 20 minutes (if you have to cook the shrimp)
Portions: 4

Ingredients:
- Farro: 1 cup (200 g or 7 oz), cooked according to instructions on package and cooled
- Shrimp: 400 g (about 14 oz), cleaned and cooked
- Cherry tomatoes: 1 cup (about 150 g or 5.3 oz), cut in half
- Fresh basil: ¼ cup (about 15 g or 0.5 oz), coarsely chopped
- Extra virgin olive oil: 3 tablespoons (45 ml)
- Lemon juice: 2 tablespoons (30 ml)
- Salt and black pepper: to taste
- Arugula: 1 cup (about 30 g or 1 oz) (optional)

Instructions:
Preparation of Farro:
- Cook farro in boiling salted water following the instructions on the package, then drain and let it cool.

Preparation of Shrimp:
- If the shrimp are not already cooked, cook them in a skillet with a drizzle of olive oil until they are pink and fully cooked.

Salad composition:
- In a large bowl, combine the cooled farro, shrimp, cherry tomatoes, basil, and arugula if using.
- In a small bowl, mix olive oil, lemon juice, salt and pepper to create the dressing.
- Pour the dressing over the salad and mix gently to blend all the ingredients.

Service:
- Let the salad rest for at least 10 minutes before serving to allow the flavors to come together.
- Taste and adjust salt and pepper if necessary.

Advice:
- For a gluten-free variation, substitute spelt for quinoa or brown rice.
- Add diced avocado or toasted pine nuts for extra creaminess and crunch.

Cold Cucumber Soup with Greek Yogurt and Dill

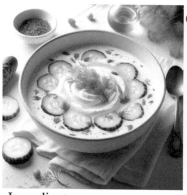

Nutritional Values per Serving:
- Calories: about 150 kcal
- Protein: 8 g
- Fat: 9 g (dependent on the oil used)
- Carbohydrates: 8 g
- Fiber: 1 g
- Sugars: 6 g

Preparation Time: 15 minutes
Cooling Time: 2 hours
Portions: 4

Ingredients:
- Cucumbers: 2 large, peeled and chopped
- Greek yogurt: 2 cups (about 480 ml)
- Fresh dill: ¼ cup (about 4 g), chopped
- Garlic: 1 clove, chopped
- Lemon juice: 2 tablespoons (30 ml)
- Cold water: 1 cup (240 ml)
- Salt and white pepper: to taste
- Extra virgin olive oil: for garnish
- Chunks of cucumber and fresh dill: for garnish

Instructions:
Soup Preparation:
- In a blender or food processor, combine chopped cucumbers, Greek yogurt, chopped dill, garlic, lemon juice, and cold water.
- Blend until smooth and creamy.
- Taste and adjust salt and pepper to suit your taste.

Cooling:
- Transfer the soup to a large bowl and cover it.
- Let cool in the refrigerator for at least 2 hours, until well chilled.

Service:
- Stir the soup well before serving.
- Pour the soup into individual bowls.
- Garnish with a drizzle of olive oil, chunks of cucumber and some fresh dill.

Advice:
- For an extra touch of flavor, add some chopped fresh mint along with the dill.
- This soup is also great served as a cold sauce for fish dishes or grilled chicken.

Salmon Burger with Fennel and Orange Salad

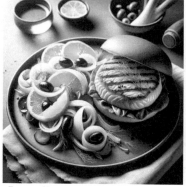

Nutritional Values per Serving:
- Calories: about 450 kcal
- Protein: 25 g
- Fat: 28 g
- Carbohydrates: 20 g
- Fiber: 5 g
- Sugars: 8 g

Preparation Time: 30 minutes
Cooking Time: 10 minutes
Portions: 4

Ingredients:
- For Salmon Burgers:
- Salmon fillets: 400 g (about 14 oz), finely chopped
- Breadcrumbs: ½ cup (about 60 g or 2.1 oz)
- Egg: 1, lightly beaten
- Chives: 2 tablespoons, chopped
- Dijon mustard: 1 teaspoon (5 ml)
- Salt and pepper: to taste
- Olive oil: for frying
- For the Fennel and Orange Salad:
- Fennel: 1 large, thinly sliced
- Oranges: 2, peeled raw and cut into slices
- Black olives: ¼ cup (about 30 g or 1 oz), pitted
- Lemon juice: 2 tablespoons (30 ml)
- Extra virgin olive oil: 3 tablespoons (45 ml
- • Salt and pepper: to taste

Instructions:
Burger Preparation:
- In a bowl, combine chopped salmon, breadcrumbs, egg, chives, Dijon mustard, salt and pepper.
- Form the mixture into 4 burgers.
- Heat olive oil in a skillet and cook the burgers for about 3-4 minutes per side until golden brown and cooked through.

Salad preparation:
- In a large bowl, combine sliced fennel, orange slices, black olives, lemon juice, and olive oil.
- Season with salt and pepper and mix gently.

Service:
- Serve the salmon burgers warm accompanied by the fennel and orange salad.

Advice:
- Add a touch of freshness to the salad with a few mint or basil leaves.
- For a gluten-free version, replace the breadcrumbs with almond flour or gluten-free breadcrumbs.

41

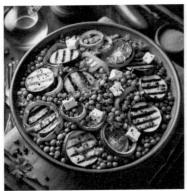

Lentil Salad with Grilled Vegetables and Crumbled Feta

Nutritional Values per Serving:
- Calories: about 350 kcal
- Protein: 18 g
- Fats: 15 g
- Carbohydrates: 40 g
- Fiber: 12 g
- Sugars: 8 g

Preparation Time: 30 minutes
Cooking Time: 15 minutes
Portions: 4

Ingredients:
- Green lentils: 1 cup (about 200 g or 7 oz), rinsed and cooked
- Zucchini: 1 large, cut into lengthwise slices
- Red peppers: 1 large, cut into wide strips
- Eggplant: 1 medium, sliced
- Red onion: 1 small, tag
- Olive oil: for grilling and seasoning
- Balsamic vinegar: 2 tablespoons (30 ml)
- Feta cheese: 100 g (about 3.5 oz), crumbled
- Fresh parsley: chopped, for garnish
- Salt and black pepper: to taste

Instructions:
Preparing Vegetables:
- Brush vegetables (zucchini, peppers, eggplant, onion) with olive oil and sprinkle lightly with salt and pepper.
- Grill vegetables on a hot grill or grill pan until they are tender and have the typical grilling stripes.

Composition of the Salad:
- In a large bowl, mix
- Add balsamic vinegar and an additional drizzle of olive oil.
- Adjust for salt and pepper.

Addition of Feta and Parsley:
- Sprinkle crumbled feta and chopped fresh parsley over the salad.

Service:
- Mix gently before serving to combine all ingredients well.
- The salad can be served lukewarm

Tips:
- For a vegan version, replace the feta with crumbled tofu or a vegan cheese.
- Add toasted nuts or seeds for a crunchy touch.

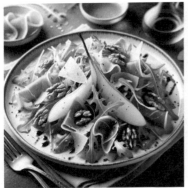

Arugula Salad with Pears, Walnuts and Bresaola

Nutritional Values per Serving:
- Calories: about 250 kcal
- Protein: 10 g
- Fats: 18 g
- Carbohydrates: 12 g
- Fiber: 3 g
- Sugars: 8 g

Preparation Time: 15 minutes
Portions: 4

Ingredients:
- Arugula: 150 g (about 5 oz)
- Pears: 2 medium-sized, thinly sliced
- Walnuts: ½ cup (about 50 g or 1.75 oz), toasted and coarsely chopped
- Bresaola: 100 g (about 3.5 oz), thinly sliced
- Parmesan cheese: flakes, to taste
- Extra virgin olive oil: 3 tablespoons (45 ml)
- Balsamic vinegar: 1 tablespoon (15 ml)
- Honey: 1 teaspoon (5 ml)
- Salt and black pepper: to taste

Instructions:
Dressing Preparation:
- In a small bowl, combine the olive oil, balsamic vinegar, honey, salt and pepper.
- Mix well until an emulsion is obtained.

Composition of the Salad:
- In a large bowl, arrange the arugula as a base.
- Add pear slices and sliced bresaola on top.
- Sprinkle with the toasted walnuts and parmesan shavings.

Seasoning and Service:
- Drizzle the prepared dressing over the salad.
- Gently stir to combine the ingredients, or let each guest season their portion as desired.

Tips:
- For an added touch of flavor, add a few drops of apple cider vinegar to the dressing.
- Bresaola can be replaced with other lean sliced meats, such as prosciutto or beef carpaccio, depending on preference.

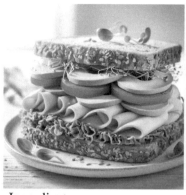

Nutritional Values per Serving:
- Calories: about 350 kcal
- Protein: 25 g
- Fats: 15 g
- Carbohydrates: 35 g
- Fiber: 8 g
- Sugars: 4 g

Preparation Time: 10 minutes
Portions: 2

Ingredients:
- Whole wheat bread: 4 slices
- Sliced turkey breast: 150 g (about 5 oz)
- Avocado: 1 ripe, sliced
- Sprouts (such as alfalfa or broccoli): 1 cup
- Light mayonnaise or Greek yogurt: 2 tablespoons (30 ml)
- Mustard: 1 teaspoon (5 ml)
- Lettuce leaves: 4
- Tomatoes: 1 medium, sliced
- Salt and black pepper: to taste

Instructions:
Bread Preparation:
- Toast the slices of whole wheat bread until they are slightly crispy.

Sandwich Assembly:
- Spread light mayonnaise or Greek yogurt on a slice of bread.
- Add a thin layer of mustard on top of the mayonnaise.

- Arrange the turkey slices on the bread.
- Add avocado slices, a pinch of salt and pepper on top of the avocado.
- Add layers of tomato and lettuce leaves.
- Complete with sprouts.
- Cover with the other slice of bread.

Service:
- Cut the sandwich diagonally and serve immediately.

Tips:
- For a lighter variation, replace the mayonnaise with hummus or another plant-based spread.
- Add slices of cucumber or red onion for an extra touch of freshness and crispness.

Chicken Wrap with Hummus, Cucumbers and Grated Carrots

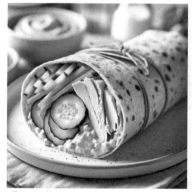

Nutritional Values per Serving:
- Calories: about 350 kcal
- Protein: 28 g
- Fats: 12 g
- Carbohydrates: 35 g
- Fiber: 6 g
- Sugars: 5 g

Preparation Time: 20 minutes
Cooking Time: 10 minutes
Portions: 4

Ingredients:
- Tortillas: 4
- Chicken breast: 2 medium, cooked and chopped or striped
- Hummus: 1 cup (about 240 ml)
- Cucumbers: 1 large, thinly sliced
- Carrots: 2 large, grated
- Lettuce leaves: 4 large
- Olive oil: for cooking
- Salt and pepper: to taste

Instructions:
Preparation of Chicken:
- Season the chicken with salt and pepper.
- Cook the chicken in a skillet with a drizzle of olive oil until golden brown and cooked through. Allow to cool and then cut into strips or shred.

Assembly of Wraps:
- Heat the tortillas slightly in a frying pan to make them more pliable.
- Spread a generous amount of hummus on each tortilla.
- Arrange the lettuce leaves on each tortilla on top of the hummus.
- Add the chicken, cucumber slices, and grated carrots.

Rolling and Service:
- • Roll the tortillas around the filling, folding the edges inward to keep the contents in.
- • Cut each wrap in half and serve, or wrap them in plastic wrap for a meal to go.

Tips:
- Vary the ingredients by adding sliced avocado or grilled red peppers for additional flavor and color.
- Experiment with different types of hummus, such as chili or olive hummus, to vary the taste.

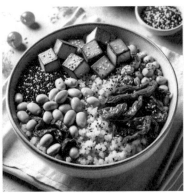

Quinoa Bowl with Edamame, Dried Tomatoes and Marinated Tofu

Nutritional Values per Serving:
- Calories: about 400 kcal
- Protein: 20 g
- Fats: 15 g
- Carbohydrates: 50 g
- Fiber: 8 g
- Sugars: 5 g

Preparation Time: 50 minutes (including marinating)
Cooking Time: 10 minutes
Portions: 2-3

Ingredients:
- Quinoa: 1 cup (about 170 g or 6 oz), cooked according to instructions on package
- Edamame: 1 cup (about 150 g or 5.3 oz), already cooked
- Dried tomatoes: ½ cup (about 75 g or 2.6 oz), chopped
- Tofu: 200 g (about 7 oz), cut into cubes
- For the tofu marinade:
- Soy sauce: 3 tablespoons (45 ml)
- Sesame oil: 1 tablespoon (15 ml)
- Garlic: 1 clove, chopped
- Maple syrup or honey: 1 teaspoon (5 ml)
- Extra virgin olive oil: for cooking
- Salt and pepper: to taste
- Sesame seeds: for garnish
- Fresh herbs (such as cilantro or parsley): chopped, for garnish

Instructions:
Tofu marinating:
- In a small bowl, combine the soy sauce, sesame oil, minced garlic, and maple syrup.
- Dip the tofu cubes into the marinade and let it sit for at least 30 minutes, preferably longer.

Tofu cooking:
- Heat some olive oil in a frying pan and cook the marinated tofu until golden brown on all sides.

Quinoa Bowl composition:
- In serving bowls, arrange a bed of cooked quinoa.
- Add edamame, sun-dried tomatoes, and marinated tofu.
- Sprinkle with sesame seeds and chopped fresh herbs.

Service:
- Serve the bowl immediately, offering extra marinade on the side if desired.

Tips:
- Vary the vegetables by adding fresh spinach or bell peppers for an extra splash of color and nutrition.
- For more intense flavor, add a tablespoon of pesto or a pinch of crushed red pepper to the marinade.

Tuna Salad with Cannellini Beans, Red Onion and Parsley

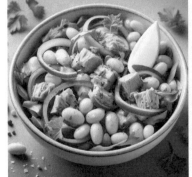

Nutritional Values per Serving:
- Calories: about 250 kcal
- Protein: 20 g
- Fats: 10 g
- Carbohydrates: 20 g
- Fiber: 5 g
- Sugars: 2 g

Preparation Time: 15 minutes
Portions: 4

Ingredients:
- Canned tuna: 200 g (about 7 oz), drained
- Cannellini beans: 1 can (400 g or 14 oz), rinsed and drained
- Red onion: 1 small, finely sliced
- Fresh parsley: ¼ cup (about 15 g), chopped
- Extra virgin olive oil: 3 tablespoons (45 ml)
- Lemon juice: 2 tablespoons (30 ml)
- Salt and black pepper: to taste

Instructions:
Preparing the Salad:
- In a large bowl, combine the drained tuna, cannellini beans, sliced red onion, and chopped parsley.

Preparation of Seasoning:
- In a small bowl, mix olive oil and lemon juice. Add salt and pepper to suit your taste.
- Pour the dressing over the salad and toss gently to combine all the ingredients well.

Service:
- Let the salad sit for at least 10 minutes before serving, allowing the flavors to meld.
- Taste and adjust salt and pepper if necessary.

Tips:
- Add taggiasca olives or capers for a touch of Mediterranean flavor.
- Serve the salad on a bed of green leaves for a more hearty and colorful meal.

Gazpacho with Shrimp and Cubed Avocado

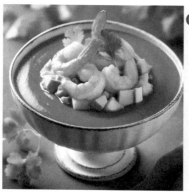

Nutritional Values per Serving:
- Calories: about 280 kcal
- Protein: 15 g
- Fats: 18 g
- Carbohydrates: 20 g
- Fiber: 5 g
- Sugars: 8 g

Preparation Time: 30 minutes
Cooling Time: 2 hours
Portions: 4

Ingredients:
- Ripe tomatoes: 6 large, peeled and chopped
- Cucumber: 1 large, peeled and chopped
- Red bell pepper: 1, chopped
- Red onion: ½, chopped
- Garlic: 2 cloves, chopped
- Red wine vinegar: 2 tablespoons (30 ml)
- Extra virgin olive oil: ¼ cup (60 ml)
- Salt and pepper: to taste
- Shrimp: 200 g (about 7 oz), cleaned and cooked
- Avocado: 1 large, ripe, diced
- Fresh coriander: for garnish

Instructions:
Preparation of Gazpacho:
- In a blender or food processor, combine the tomatoes, cucumber, red bell pepper, onion, garlic, red wine vinegar, and olive oil.
- Blend until smooth.
- Taste and adjust salt and pepper.
- Let cool in the refrigerator for at least 2 hours, or until well chilled.

Preparation of Shrimp and Avocado:
- Just before serving, cook the shrimp in a skillet with a drizzle of olive oil until pink and cooked through.
- Cut the avocado into cubes.

Service:
- Pour cold gazpacho into bowls.
- Add cooked shrimp and avocado cubes to the top of each serving.
- Garnish with fresh chopped cilantro.

Tips:
- For a spicy note, add a chopped fresh chili pepper to the mixture before blending.
- Serve the gazpacho with crusty bread croutons for added texture.

Cold Tomato Soup with Basil and Wholewheat Croutons

Nutritional Values per Serving:
- Calories: about 200 kcal
- Protein: 4 g
- Fats: 10 g
- Carbohydrates: 25 g
- Fiber: 5 g
- Sugars: 10 g

Preparation Time: 15 minutes
Cooling Time: 2 hours
Portions: 4

Ingredients:
- Ripe tomatoes: 6 large, chopped
- Red onion: 1 medium, chopped
- Cucumber: 1 small, peeled and chopped
- Red bell pepper: 1, chopped
- Garlic: 2 cloves, chopped
- Fresh basil: 1 handful, chopped, plus extra for garnish
- Red wine vinegar: 2 tablespoons (30 ml)
- Extra virgin olive oil: ¼ cup (60 ml)
- Salt and pepper: to taste
- Whole wheat bread: 4 slices, toasted and cut into cubes

Instructions:
Soup Preparation:
- In a blender or food processor, combine the tomatoes, onion, cucumber, bell bell pepper, garlic, and most of the basil. Blend until smooth.
- Add the red wine vinegar and olive oil and blend again until the soup is smooth.
- Taste and adjust for salt and pepper.
- Let cool in the refrigerator for at least 2 hours.

Preparing Crostini:
- Toast the slices of whole wheat bread, then cut them into cubes.

Service:
- Serve the soup cold in bowls.
- Add whole-wheat bread croutons and garnish with the remaining chopped fresh basil.

Tips:
- Add a tablespoon of sour cream or Greek yogurt for a creamier variation.
- For a spicy touch, add a chopped red chili pepper while preparing the soup.

Vegetarian Quinoa and Pea Burger with Mixed Salad

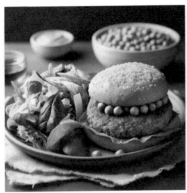

Nutritional Values per Serving:
- Calories: about 300 kcal
- Protein: 12 g
- Fats: 15 g
- Carbohydrates: 30 g
- Fiber: 6 g
- Sugars: 3 g

Preparation Time: 45 minutes
Cooking Time: 10 minutes
Portions: 4

Ingredients:
- Quinoa: ½ cup (about 85 g or 3 oz), cooked and cooled
- Peas: 1 cup (about 150 g or 5.3 oz), cooked and mashed
- Breadcrumbs: ½ cup (about 60 g or 2.1 oz)
- Egg: 1, for binding (optional, can be omitted for a vegan version)
- Onion: 1 small, finely chopped
- Garlic: 2 cloves, chopped
- Coriander or parsley
- Smoked paprika: 1 teaspoon (5 ml)
- Salt and pepper: to taste
- Olive oil: for cooking
- Mixed salad: 2 cups (about 50 g or 1.75 oz), such as lettuce, arugula, and spinach
- Salad dressing: olive oil, balsamic vinegar, salt and pepper

Instructions:
Burger Preparation:
- In a large bowl, mix cooked quinoa, crushed peas, bread crumbs, egg (if using), onion, garlic, cilantro or parsley, paprika, salt and pepper until smooth.
- Form the mixture into 4 burgers and let stand for about 30 minutes in the refrigerator to firm up.

Burger Cooking:
- Heat olive oil in a nonstick skillet and cook the burgers for 4-5 minutes per side, until golden brown and cooked through.

Preparing the Salad:
- In a bowl, mix the mixed salad with a little olive oil, balsamic vinegar, salt and pepper.

Service:
- Serve the burgers hot accompanied by the mixed salad.

Tips:
- Add avocado slices or a tahini sauce to further enrich the burger.
- Experiment with different kinds of herbs and spices to vary the flavor of the burgers.

Thai Chicken Salad with Cucumbers, Carrots and Peanut Sauce

Nutritional Values per Serving:
- Calories: about 350 kcal
- Protein: 28 g
- Fats: 18 g
- Carbohydrates: 18 g
- Fiber: 4 g
- Sugars: 8 g

Preparation Time: 20 minutes
Portions: 4

Ingredients:
- Chicken breast: 2 medium, cooked and shredded
- Cucumbers: 2 medium, cut into julienne strips
- Carrots: 2 large, cut into julienne strips
- Fresh cilantro: ¼ cup, chopped
- Roasted peanuts: ¼ cup, coarsely chopped
- For the Peanut Sauce:
- Peanut butter: 3 tablespoons (45 ml)
- Hot water: 2 tablespoons (30 ml) to dilute
- Soy sauce: 1 tablespoon (15 ml)
- Lime juice: 1 tablespoon (15 ml)
- Honey: 1 teaspoon (5 ml)
- Garlic: 1 clove, chopped
- Crushed red chili pepper: 1 teaspoon (5 ml) (optional)

Instructions:
Preparation of Peanut Sauce:
- In a small bowl, mix peanut butter with hot water until smooth.
- Add soy sauce, lime juice, honey, minced garlic, and red chili. Mix well until all ingredients are combined.

Salad composition:
- In a large bowl, combine shredded chicken, cucumbers, carrots, cilantro, and chopped peanuts.
- Pour the peanut sauce over the salad and toss gently to evenly coat the ingredients.

Service:
- Serve the salad immediately, garnished with additional chopped peanuts and fresh cilantro if desired.

Tips:
- Add diced fresh mango or red bell pepper strips for a touch of sweetness and color.
- The peanut sauce can be customized according to personal taste by adding more or less honey, lime juice or chili.

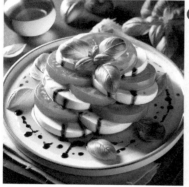

Caprese Salad with Buffalo Mozzarella, Tomatoes and Basil

Nutritional Values per Serving:
- Calories: about 300 kcal
- Protein: 18 g
- Fat: 22 g (dependent on the oil used)
- Carbohydrates: 6 g
- Fiber: 2 g
- Sugars: 4 g

Preparation Time: 10 minutes
Portions: 2-3

Ingredients:
- Low-fat cottage cheese: 200 g (about 7 oz), cut into thick slices
- Ripe tomatoes: 3 large, cut into thick slices
- Fresh basil: 1 handful of leaves
- Extra virgin olive oil: 3 tablespoons (45 ml)
- Salt and black pepper: to taste
- Balsamic vinegar: optional, for garnish

Instructions:
Preparation:
- Arrange tomato and mozzarella slices alternately on a serving plate.
- Insert fresh basil leaves between the tomato and mozzarella slices.

Seasoning:
- Drizzle extra virgin olive oil over the tomato and mozzarella slices.
- Sprinkle lightly with salt and freshly ground black pepper.
- If desired, add a drizzle of balsamic vinegar for a touch of sweet acidity.

Service:
- Serve the salad immediately to enjoy the freshness of its ingredients.

Tips:
- For an extra touch, add black olives or capers.
- Keep ingredients cool until serving to maintain freshness.

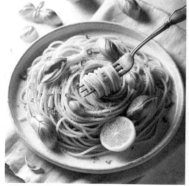

Spaghetti Integral with Lemon and Basil

Nutritional Values per Serving:
- Calories: about 400 kcal
- Protein: 14 g
- Fats: 14 g
- Carbohydrates: 58 g
- Fiber: 8 g
- Sugars: 2 g

Preparation Time: 20 minutes
Cooking Time: 10 minutes
Portions: 4

Ingredients:
- Whole wheat spaghetti: 400 g (about 14 oz)
- Lemons: 2, the grated zest and juice
- Fresh basil: 1 handful, chopped
- Garlic: 2 cloves, finely chopped
- Red pepper: 1 small, chopped (optional)
- Extra virgin olive oil: ¼ cup (60 ml)
- Salt and black pepper: to taste
- Parmesan cheese: for garnish, grated

Instructions:
Cooking Pasta:
- Bring a large pot of salted water to a boil. Cook whole wheat spaghetti according to the instructions on the package until al dente.
- Drain the pasta, reserving some of the cooking water.

Preparation of Seasoning:
- While the pasta is cooking, heat olive oil in a large skillet over medium heat.
- Add minced garlic (and chili, if using) and sauté for about 1 minute, until golden brown.
- Remove from heat and add lemon zest and juice.

Finish:
- Add the cooked spaghetti to the pan with the oil and lemon.
- Add chopped basil and mix well. If necessary, add a little pasta cooking water to create a light emulsion.
- Season with salt and pepper to taste.

Service:
- Serve the spaghetti hot, garnished with grated parmesan cheese.

Tips:
- Add sautéed shrimp or grilled chicken for a higher protein version.
- Experiment by adding other herbs such as thyme or parsley to vary the taste.

Pocket Pita with Hummus, Grilled Vegetables and Feta Cheese

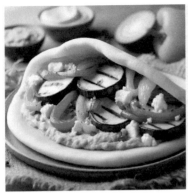

Nutritional Values per Serving:
- Calories: about 350 kcal
- Protein: 12 g
- Fats: 18 g
- Carbohydrates: 35 g
- Fiber: 5 g
- Sugars: 6 g

Preparation Time: 30 minutes
Cooking Time: 15 minutes
Portions: 4

Ingredients:
- Peter: 4 sandwiches
- Hummus: 1 cup (about 240 ml)
- Zucchini: 2 medium-sized, sliced lengthwise
- Peppers: 2 (one red and one yellow), cut into strips
- Red onion: 1 large, sliced
- Feta cheese: 100 g (about 3.5 oz), crumbled
- Olive oil: for grilling
- Salt and pepper: to taste

Instructions:
Grilling Vegetables:
- Preheat a grill or grill pan.
- Grease the zucchini, bell bell pepper and onion slices with olive oil and sprinkle lightly with salt and pepper.
- Grill the vegetables until they are soft and have grill marks, turning them once for even cooking.

Pita preparation:
- Cut the pita sandwiches in half to form pockets.
- Spread a generous amount of hummus inside each pita pocket.

Assembly:
- Fill each pita with the grilled vegetables.
- Add crumbled feta cheese on top of the vegetables.

Service:
- Serve the pita immediately while the vegetables are still warm.

Tips:
- For a spicy touch, add a few slices of fresh chili or a splash of hot sauce to the filling.
- Vary the vegetables according to the season to keep the dish fresh and interesting.

Spaghetti with Creamy Roasted Peppers

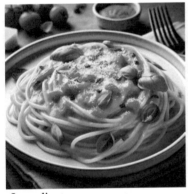

Nutritional Values per Serving:
- Calories: about 550 kcal
- Protein: 17 g
- Fats: 20 g
- Carbohydrates: 75 g
- Fiber: 6 g
- Sugars: 8 g

Preparation Time: 45 minutes
Cooking Time: 30 minutes
Portions: 4

Advice:
- For a vegan version, substitute Parmesan cheese for grated vegan cheese.
- Add capers or olives for an extra touch of Mediterranean flavor.

Ingredients:
- Spaghetti: 400 g (about 14 oz)
- Red peppers: 3 large
- Garlic: 2 cloves, chopped
- Onion: 1 medium, chopped
- Soy or oat cream: 100 ml (about 3.4 fl oz)
- Extra virgin olive oil: 3 tablespoons (45 ml)
- Salt and pepper: to taste
- Fresh basil: for garnish
- Parmesan cheese: for garnish, grated

Instructions:
Roasting Peppers:
- Preheat the oven to 200°C (about 400°F).
- Cut the peppers in half, remove seeds and ribs, and arrange them on a baking sheet with the skin side up.
- Roast in the oven until the skin turns black and blistered, about 15-20 minutes.
- Remove the peppers from the oven, cover them with aluminum foil or place them in a plastic bag for 10 minutes (this will help peel them easily).
- Peel off the burned skin and coarsely chop the pulp.

Preparation of the Sauce:
- In a large skillet, heat olive oil and sauté onion and garlic until soft and translucent.
- Add chopped peppers and cook for a few minutes.
- Transfer to a blender, add the cream, and blend until smooth.
- Return the sauce to the pan, heat over medium heat, and season with salt and pepper.

Cooking Pasta:
- Cook spaghetti in a pot of boiling salted water until al dente.
- Drain the pasta, reserving some of the cooking water.

Finish and Service:
- Add the spaghetti to the bell pepper sauce in the skillet.
- Mix well, adding a little cooking water if necessary to make the sauce more fluid.
- Serve hot, garnished with chopped fresh basil and Parmesan cheese.

Protein Penne with Avocado Sauce

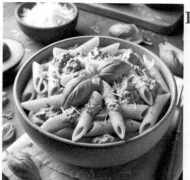

Nutritional Values per Serving:
- Calories: about 500 kcal
- Protein: 25 g
- Fats: 20 g
- Carbohydrates: 60 g
- Fiber: 8 g
- Sugars: 2 g

Preparation Time: 20 minutes
Cooking Time: 10 minutes
Portions: 4

Ingredients:
- Protein Penne: 400 g (about 14 oz)
- Ripe avocados: 2
- Garlic: 1 clove, chopped
- Lemon juice: 2 tablespoons (30 ml)
- Extra virgin olive oil: 2 tablespoons (30 ml)
- Chili flakes: 1 teaspoon (optional)
- Salt and black pepper: to taste
- Parmesan cheese: for garnish, grated
- Fresh basil leaves: for garnish

Instructions:
Cooking Pasta:
- Bring a large pot of salted water to a boil. Cook the penne according to the instructions on the package until they are al dente.
- Drain the pasta, reserving a cup of the cooking water.

Preparation of Avocado Sauce:
- In a blender, combine peeled and pitted avocados, garlic, lemon juice, olive oil, chili, salt and pepper.
- Blend until smooth. If the sauce is too thick, add a little of the pasta cooking water to achieve the desired consistency.

Finish and Service:
- In a large bowl, mix the penne with the avocado sauce until well seasoned.
- Serve the penne hot, garnished with grated Parmesan cheese and fresh basil leaves.

Advice:
- Add chunks of fresh tomato or olives for an extra touch of freshness and flavor.
- For a vegan option, substitute parmesan cheese for grated vegan cheese or nutritional yeast flakes.

In conclusion, this collection of 30 recipes for lunch at work is designed to provide balanced, nutritious and tasty meals. Although not all of the recipes are ideal for bringing to work due to various logistical requirements, each is designed to be easy to prepare and, in most cases, easy to transport and consume without the need for heating.

Cold salads and soups, for example, offer a refreshing way to incorporate a variety of vegetables, lean proteins, and healthy fats. On the other hand, veggie wraps and burgers provide hearty alternatives rich in fiber and vitamins, ideal for a satiating lunch.

Each recipe includes details on preparation time, difficulty and nutritional values per serving, allowing you to choose and plan your meals according to your personal needs and preferences. It is essential to remember that maintaining a varied and balanced diet is crucial to preserving health and ensuring a constant level of energy while working.

Experimenting with different combinations of ingredients and flavors can not only make meals more interesting, but also help you stay motivated and fulfilled by your food choices.

Enjoy your meal and enjoy your work!

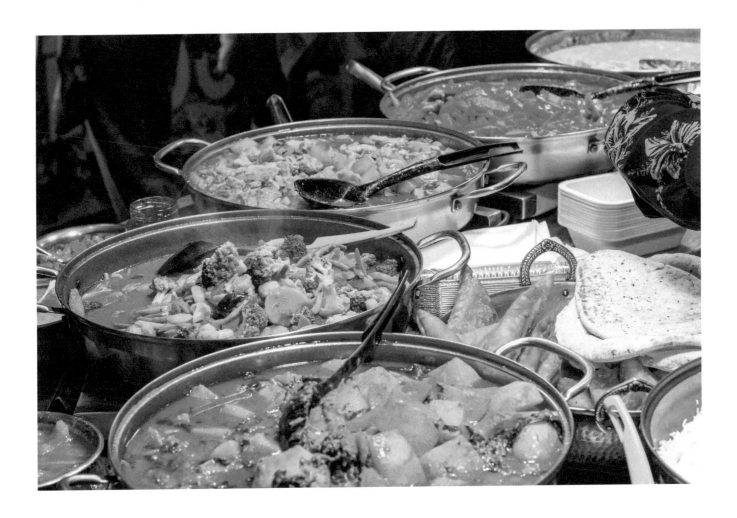

CHAPTER 9: THE SUPPER - AN OPPORTUNITY TO NOURISH AND HEAL THE LIVER

9.1 Recipes for Dinner

Introduction to Evening Meal

Dinner is more than just a meal; it is an opportunity to nourish the body and support the liver's vital role after a busy day. The liver, a powerhouse organ, performs multiple detoxification and metabolism functions overnight. Choosing foods that support these processes is crucial without overloading the organ.

Principles for a Liver-Beneficial Dinner

- Lightness: An evening meal should be manageable; excessive portions can overload the liver at night.
- Nutritional Balance: Incorporates a good source of lean protein, complex carbohydrates from vegetables and whole grains, and healthy fats to promote satiety and optimization of liver function.
- Low in Saturated Fats and Sugars: Limit foods high in saturated fats and simple sugars, which can contribute to fat accumulation in the liver and insulin resistance.

Baked cod steak with cherry tomatoes and olives

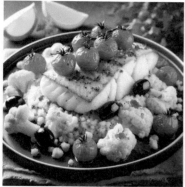

Nutritional Values per Serving:
- Calories: about 250 kcal
- Protein: 27 g
- Fats: 8 g
- Carbohydrates: 15 g
- Fiber: 3 g
- Sugars: 4 g

Preparation Time: 10 minutes
Cooking Time: 25 minutes
Serving Size: 4

Ingredients:
- Cod: 4 slices
- Cherry tomatoes: (200 g, about 7 oz), cut in half
- Black olives: (50 g, about 1,7 oz) pitted and chopped
- Cauliflower: 1 large, grated to make couscous
- Olive oil: for seasoning
- Salt and pepper: to taste
- Lemon: 1, the juice
- Parsley: chopped, for garnish
- **Instructions:**

Preparation of Cod:
- Preheat the oven to 200°C.
- Arrange the cod slices on a baking sheet lined with parchment paper.
- Season with salt, pepper and a drizzle of olive oil.
- Scatter the cherry tomatoes and olives around the fish.
- Bake for 15-20 minutes or until cooked through.

Cauliflower Couscous:
- Use a food processor to grate the cauliflower to a couscous-like consistency.
- Heat a drizzle of oil in a frying pan and saute for 5-8 minutes. Season with salt and pepper.

Service:
- Arrange the cooked cod on a serving plate.
- Accompany with cauliflower couscous.
- Drizzle the fish with lemon juice and garnish with chopped parsley.

Advice:
- Add capers or anchovies for an extra touch of Mediterranean flavor.
- Serve with a slice of lemon to add a touch of freshness.

Roasted chicken breast with citrus sauce

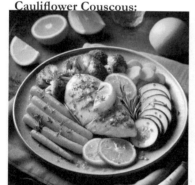

Nutritional Values per Serving:
- Calories: about 350 kcal
- Protein: 35 g
- Fats: 15 g
- Carbohydrates: 10 g
- Fiber: 3 g
- Sugars: 7 g

Preparation Time: 30 minutes
Cooking Time: 25 minutes
Serving Size: 4

Ingredients:
- Roast chicken breast: 4 breasts
- Lemons: 2, the juice and zest
- Oranges: 2, the juice and zest
- Garlic: 2 cloves, chopped
- Honey: 1 tablespoon
- Rosemary: 1 sprig, chopped
- Olive oil: for cooking
- Salt and pepper: to taste
- Mixed vegetables (carrots, broccoli, zucchini): (400 g, about 14 oz) cut into pieces**Instructions:**

Preparation of the Sauce:
- Mix the juice and zest of lemons and oranges with garlic, honey and rosemary in a bowl.

Marinating Chicken:
- Marina the chicken breasts with half the citrus sauce for at least 1 hour.

Cooking the Chicken:
- Heat oil in a skillet and brown the marinated chicken until golden brown.
- Bake at 200°C for 20 minutes or until cooked through.

Preparing Vegetables:
- Steam the vegetables until they are tender but still crisp.

Service:
- Serve the roasted chicken with the steamed vegetables.
- Nestle it with the rest of the citrus sauce.
- Garnish with additional citrus zest if desired.

Advice:
- For a crispier crust on chicken, use the oven's grill function during the last 5 minutes of cooking.
- Add a pinch of chili flakes to the sauce for a spicy touch.

Stuffed zucchini with brown rice, tomatoes and herbs.

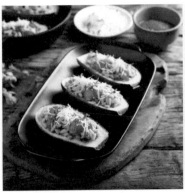

Nutritional Values per Serving:
- Calories: about 220 kcal
- Protein: 8 g
- Fats: 10 g
- Carbohydrates: 27 g
- Fiber: 4 g
- Sugars: 5 g

Preparation Time: 15 minutes
Cooking Time: 30 minutes
Serving Size: 4

Advice:
- Vary the herbs according to availability or personal preference to diversify the taste.
- Add protein such as ground meat or crumbled tofu to the filling for a more substantial meal.

Ingredients:
- Zucchini: 4 medium-sized, cut in half lengthwise and hollowed out
- Brown rice: 1 cup (about 185 g, 6,5 oz), cooked
- Tomatoes: 2 medium, chopped
- Onion: 1 small, chopped
- Garlic: 2 cloves, chopped
- Herbs (basil, parsley, thyme): 2 tablespoons, chopped
- Olive oil: 2 tablespoons
- Salt and pepper: to taste
- Parmesan cheese: (50 g, about1,7 oz) grated
- **Instructions:**

Preparing Zucchini:
- Preheat the oven to 190°C.
- Hollow out the inside of the zucchini, leaving a thickness of about 1 cm.
- Mince the removed pulp and set it aside.

Preparing the Stuffing:
- In a skillet, heat olive oil and sauté the onion and garlic until transparent.
- Add zucchini flesh, rice, tomatoes, and herbs. Cook for about 5 minutes.
- Season with salt and pepper.

Stuffing Zucchini:
- Fills the zucchini boats with the rice mix.
- Sprinkle grated Parmesan cheese on top.

Cooking:
- Place the zucchini in a baking dish and bake for 20-25 minutes, until the zucchini is tender and the cheese is golden brown.

Service:
- Serve hot, garnished with additional fresh herbs if desired.

Pesto zucchini noodles with shrimp

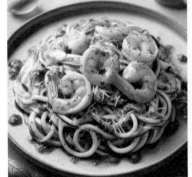

Nutritional Values per Serving:
- Calories: about 280 kcal
- Protein: 24 g
- Fats: 12 g
- Carbohydrates: 10 g
- Fiber: 2 g
- Sugars: 4 g

Preparation Time: 10 minutes
Cooking Time: 10 minutes
Portions: 4

Ingredients:
- Zucchini: 4 large, cut into noodles with a spiralizer
- Shrimps: (300 g, about 10,5 oz) shelled and cleaned
- Pesto: 120 ml (about ½ cup)
- Garlic: 2 cloves, chopped
- Olive oil: 2 tablespoons
- Salt and pepper: to taste
- Lemon: 1, the juice for seasoning
- Parmesan cheese: for garnish, grated
- Fresh basil: for garnish

Instructions:

Preparation of Shrimp:
- In a large frying pan, heat 1 tablespoon of olive oil.
- Add minced garlic and sauté briefly until fragrant.
- Add shrimp and cook until pink and opaque, about 3-4 minutes. Season with salt and pepper.
- Remove the shrimp from the pan and set aside.

Cooking Spaghetti Squash:
- In the same pan, add the remaining oil and the zucchini noodles.
- Saute them for 2-3 minutes, until just tender.

Assembly:
- Reduce the heat and add the pesto to the zucchini noodles, stirring to coat evenly.
- Add the cooked shrimp and stir gently to combine.
- Season with lemon juice and adjust salt and pepper if necessary.

Service:
- Serve the spaghetti hot, garnished with chopped fresh basil and grated Parmesan cheese.

Advice:
- For a richer dish, you can toast some pine nuts and add them to the dish before serving.
- If you prefer a less caloric pesto, consider making a version with less oil or with added Greek yogurt to maintain the creaminess.

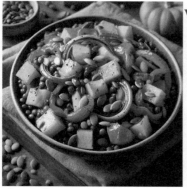

Warm lentil salad with roasted vegetables and pumpkin seeds.

Nutritional Values per Serving:
- Calories: about 280 kcal
- Protein: 14 g
- Fats: 9 g
- Carbohydrates: 35 g
- Fiber: 8 g
- Sugars: 5 g

Preparation Time: 15 minutes
Cooking Time: 55 minutes
Serving Size: 4

Ingredients:
- Lentils: 200 g (approximately 7.05 oz), rinsed and drained
- Pumpkin: 200 g (approximately 7.05 oz), diced
- Bell peppers: 1 red, 1 yellow, cut into pieces
- Red onion: 1, cut into wedges
- Pumpkin seeds: 30 g (approximately 1.06 oz), toasted
- Olive oil: for roasting and dressing
- Balsamic vinegar: 2 tablespoons
- Salt and pepper: to taste
- Herbs (rosemary, thyme): chopped, 1 tablespoon

Instructions:
Cooking Lentils:
- Cook lentils in boiling water for 20-25 minutes until tender. Drain and set aside.

Roasting Vegetables:
- Preheat the oven to 200°C.
- Arrange squash, peppers and onion on a baking sheet, season with oil, salt, pepper and herbs.
- Roast for 25-30 minutes until they are caramelized and tender.

Salad Assembly:
- In a large bowl, mix the hot lentils with the roasted vegetables.
- Add toasted pumpkin seeds and season with balsamic vinegar and an additional drizzle of olive oil.

Service:
- Serve the salad warm, adjusting salt and pepper if necessary.

Advice:
- For an extra crunch, add toasted walnuts or slivered almonds.
- A squeeze of fresh lemon juice can add a lively freshness before serving.

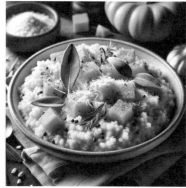

Quinoa risotto with pumpkin and parmesan cheese

Nutrition Values per Serving:
- Calories: about 280 kcal
- Protein: 10 g
- Fats: 9 g
- Carbohydrates: 40 g
- Fiber: 5 g
- Sugars: 3 g

Preparation Time: 10 minutes
Cooking Time: 30 minutes
Portions: 4

Ingredients:
- Quinoa: (200 g, about 7 oz) rinsed
- Pumpkin: (300 g, about 10,5 oz) diced
- Vegetable broth: (500 ml, about 17 fl oz)
- Onion: 1 small, chopped
- Garlic: 1 clove, chopped
- Parmesan cheese: (50 g, about 1,7oz) grated (optional, use a low-fat version if available)
- Extra virgin olive oil: 2 tablespoons
- Sage: a few leaves, chopped
- Salt and pepper: to taste
- **Instructions:**

Preparing Pumpkin:
- In a frying pan, heat a tablespoon of extra virgin olive oil over medium heat.
- Add squash and saute until lightly browned and tender, about 10 minutes. Remove and set aside.

Cooking Quinoa:
- In the same pan, add the remaining tablespoon of oil.
- Fry the onion and garlic until they become transparent.
- Add the quinoa and let it toast for a couple of minutes.
- Gradually pour in the vegetable broth, continuing to stir, until the quinoa is cooked and creamy, about 15 to 20 minutes.

Assembly:
- Once the quinoa is cooked, incorporate the roasted squash.
- Add grated Parmesan cheese, chopped sage, and season with salt and pepper.
- Mix well until all ingredients are hot and well combined.

Service:
- Serve the risotto hot, garnished with an additional sprinkling of Parmesan cheese and fresh sage leaves if desired.

Advice:
- For a completely vegan version, eliminate the parmesan cheese or replace it with a grated vegan alternative.
- Add toasted walnuts for a crunchy touch and additional healthy fats.

Salmon fillet with mustard and honey sauce

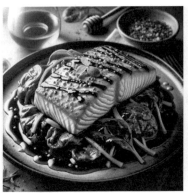

Nutrition Values per Serving:
- Calories: about 320 kcal
- Protein: 23 g
- Fats: 15 g
- Carbohydrates: 10 g
- Fiber: 2 g
- Sugars: 8 g

Preparation Time: 10 minutes
Cooking Time: 15 minutes
Portions: 4

Ingredients:
- Salmon fillets: 4 (about 150 g, 5,30 oz each)
- Honey: 2 tablespoons
- Dijon mustard: 1 tablespoon
- Extra virgin olive oil: for cooking
- Lemon: 1, the juice
- Fresh spinach: (400 g, about 14 oz)
- Garlic: 1 clove, chopped
- Salt and pepper: to taste

Instructions:
Preparation of Mustard and Honey Sauce:
- In a small bowl, mix well the honey, Dijon mustard, and lemon juice. Set aside.

Cooking Salmon:
- Preheat the oven to 200°C.
- Season the salmon fillets with salt and pepper and a drizzle of extra virgin olive oil.
- Arrange the salmon on a baking sheet lined with parchment paper.
- Brush the salmon with the mustard and honey sauce.
- Bake for 12 to 15 minutes, or until salmon is cooked to your liking.

Cooking Spinach:
- While the salmon is in the oven, heat a drizzle of extra virgin olive oil in a large skillet over medium-high heat.
- Add minced garlic and sauté briefly until fragrant.
- Add spinach and cook, stirring, until wilted and tender.
- Season with salt and pepper to taste.

Service:
- Serve the cooked salmon fillets with the sautéed spinach on the side.
- Drizzle the salmon with the remaining mustard and honey sauce, if desired.

Advice:
- For an extra touch, add a pinch of chili flakes to the spinach as it cooks for a spicier flavor.
- A sprinkling of toasted sesame seeds over the salmon can add crunch and flavor.

Lean beef stew with root vegetables and a touch of rosemary

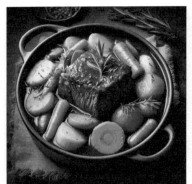

Nutritional Values per Serving:
- Calories: about 350 kcal
- Protein: 35 g
- Fats: 15 g
- Carbohydrates: 15 g
- Fiber: 3 g
- Sugars: 5 g

Preparation Time: 20 minutes
Cooking Time: 1 hour and 30 minutes
Portions: 4

Ingredients:
- Whole wheat pizza crust: 1 large
- Tomato sauce: (200 ml, 6.76 fl oz (0.85 cups)
- Arugula: (100 g, 3.53 oz)
- Parmigiano-Reggiano cheese: (50g, 1.76 oz, shaved)
- Extra virgin olive oil: to taste
- Garlic: 1 clove, minced
- Salt and pepper: to taste

Instructions:
Browning of Beef:
- Heat extra virgin olive oil in a large saucepan over medium-high heat.
- Add the beef cubes and brown them until nicely browned on all sides.

Addition of the Vegetables and Flavors:
- Turn the heat down to medium and add the onion and garlic, frying them until they become transparent.
- Incorporate root vegetables and rosemary sprigs, stirring to blend flavors.

Cooking the Stew:
- Pour the beef broth into the saucepan, making sure it completely covers the ingredients.
- Bring to a boil, then reduce heat and let simmer covered for about 1-1.5 hours, or until beef and vegetables are tender.
- Taste and adjust for salt and pepper.

Service:
- Remove the rosemary sprigs before serving.
- Serve the stew hot, ideal for a cold day.

Advice:
- For a richer flavor, you can add a splash of red wine while cooking and let it evaporate before adding the broth.
- A pinch of freshly ground black pepper or chili flakes can add a pleasant heat to the dish.

Pizza on whole wheat flour base with tomato

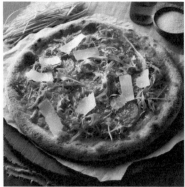

Nutritional Values per Serving:
- Calories: about 300 kcal
- Protein: 12 g
- Fats: 10 g
- Carbohydrates: 40 g
- Fiber: 5 g
- Sugars: 4 g

Preparation Time: 15 minutes
Cooking Time: 12 minutes
Serving Size: 4

Ingredients:
- Whole wheat flour pizza base: 1 large
- Tomato puree: (250 ml, 8.45 fl oz (1.06 cups)
- Arugula: (100 g, 3,53 oz)
- Parmesan cheese: (50 g, 1,76 oz) in flakes
- Extra virgin olive oil: for seasoning
- Garlic: 1 clove, chopped
- Salt and pepper: to taste

Instructions:
Preparation of the Base:
- Preheat the oven to 220°C.
- Spread the pizza base on a baking sheet lined with parchment paper.

Preparation of Seasoning:
- In a small bowl, mix tomato puree with minced garlic, salt and pepper.
- Spread the sauce evenly over the pizza base.

Pizza Cooking:
- Bake the base with sauce in the preheated oven for about 10 to 12 minutes, until the edges turn golden and crisp.

Adding the arugula and Parmesan cheese:
- Remove the pizza from the oven and spread the fresh arugula evenly on top.
- Add parmesan cheese flakes and a drizzle of extra virgin olive oil.

Service:
- Serve the pizza immediately, adding additional parmesan shavings or a pinch of fresh black pepper if desired.

Advice:
- For a richer variation, you can add thin slices of prosciutto before adding the arugula.
- Consider adding taggiasca olives or capers for a touch of Mediterranean flavor.

Vegetable pad thai with tofu and rice noodles

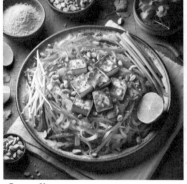

Nutritional Values per Serving:
- Calories: about 350 kcal
- Protein: 12 g
- Fats: 10 g
- Carbohydrates: 50 g
- Fiber: 4 g
- Sugars: 8 g

Preparation Time: 15 minutes
Cooking Time: 20 minutes
Serving Size: 4
Advice:
- For more intense flavor, add a tablespoon of tamarind paste to the sauce.
- Vary the vegetables according to the season to keep the dish fresh and interesting.

Ingredients:
- Rice noodles: (200 g, about 7 oz)
- Tofu: (200 g, about 7 oz) cut into cubes
- Carrots: 2 medium, cut into julienne strips
- Peppers: 1 red, cut into strips
- Green onion: 3, chopped
- Garlic: 2 cloves, chopped
- Peanuts: (30 g, about 1 oz) chopped
- Egg: 1, beaten (optional, can be omitted for a vegan version)
- Extra virgin olive oil: 2 tablespoons
- Soy sauce: 3 tablespoons
- Lime juice: 2 tablespoons
- Coconut sugar: 1 tablespoon
- Soybean sprouts: a handful
- Fresh coriander: for garnish
- Fresh red chili pepper: chopped, for garnish (optional)

Instructions:
Preparation of Noodles:
- Cook the rice noodles according to the instructions on the package, then drain and set aside.

Tofu preparation:
- In a large frying pan or wok, heat a tablespoon of extra virgin olive oil.
- Add tofu and saute until golden brown and crispy. Remove and set aside.

Cooking Vegetables:
- In the same wok, add the remaining oil and sauté the garlic, green onion, peppers, and carrots until tender.

Adding the Remaining Ingredients:
- Add the egg to the center of the wok and stir quickly until cooked.
- Add the noodles, tofu, soy sauce, lime juice, and coconut sugar.
- Mix well to combine all ingredients.

Service:
- Serve Pad Thai hot, garnished with chopped peanuts, soybean sprouts, fresh cilantro, and red chili pepper, if used.

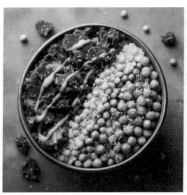

Buddha bowl with barley, chickpea r Toasti, kale and tahini dressing.

Nutrition Values per Serving:
- Calories: about 300 kcal
- Protein: 12 g
- Fats: 10 g
- Carbohydrates: 40 g
- Fiber: 8 g
- Sugars: 4 g

Preparation Time: 20 minutes
Cooking Time: 10 minutes
Portions: 4

Ingredients:
- Barley: 200 g, 7.05 oz, cooked
- Chickpeas: 200g, 7.05 oz, drained and toasted
- Kale: 150g, 5.29 oz, chopped
- Tahini dressing: 3 tablespoons
- Lemon: 1, juiced
- Garlic: 1 clove, minced
- Extra virgin olive oil: to taste
- Salt and pepper: to taste
- Sesame seeds: for garnish

Instructions:
Preparation of Roasted Chickpeas:
- Heat a skillet over medium-high heat and toast the chickpeas with a little oil until crisp, about 10 minutes. Season with salt and pepper.

Preparation of Curly Cabbage:
- In a large bowl, massage chopped kale with a little oil and lemon juice until softened.

Preparing Tahini Dressing:
- In a small bowl, mix tahini, minced garlic, remaining lemon juice, and enough water to make a smooth, pourable consistency. Season with salt and pepper to taste.

Assembly of the Buddha Bowl:
- Arrange the cooked barley as a base in the bowl.
- Add roasted chickpeas and kale.
- Pour the tahini dressing over the top.
- Garnish with sesame seeds.

Advice:
- To add additional flavor and color, include grated carrots or chopped raw beets.
- For a spicy touch, add some chili flakes to the tahini dressing.

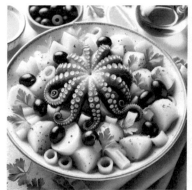

Octopus salad with potatoes, celery and olives

Nutritional Values per Serving:
- Calories: about 250 kcal
- Protein: 20 g
- Fats: 15 g
- Carbohydrates: 10 g
- Fiber: 2 g
- Sugars: 1 g

Preparation Time: 15 minutes
Cooking Time: 0 minutes (if the octopus is already precooked)
Portions: 4

Ingredients:
- Octopus: (300 g, 10.5 oz) precooked and cut into pieces
- Potatoes: (200 g, about 7 oz) boiled and diced
- Celery: (100 g, about 3.5) chopped
- Black olives: (50 g, about 1.7oz) pitted
- Lemon: 1, the juice and zest
- Extra virgin olive oil: 3 tablespoons
- Salt and pepper: to taste
- Fresh parsley: chopped, for garnish

Instructions:
Salad preparation:
- In a large bowl, combine pre-cooked octopus, boiled potatoes, chopped celery, and black olives.

Seasoning:
- In a small bowl, mix lemon juice and zest with extra virgin olive oil.
- Season with salt and pepper according to taste.

Assembly:
- Pour the dressing over the octopus and vegetable mixture.
- Mix well to ensure that everything is evenly seasoned.

Service:
- Transfer the salad to serving plates.
- Garnish with fresh chopped parsley before serving.

Advice:
- For an extra touch of flavor, add a pinch of chili flakes or capers to the dressing.
- Be sure to cool the potatoes and octopus before mixing them with the other ingredients to maintain the freshness of the salad.

Vegetarian chili with black beans, corn and peppers

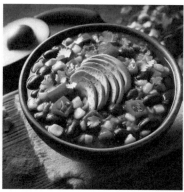

Nutritional Values per Serving:
- Calories: about 300 kcal
- Protein: 15 g
- Fats: 10 g
- Carbohydrates: 40 g
- Fiber: 12 g
- Sugars: 8 g

Preparation Time: 15 minutes
Cooking Time: 45 minutes
Serving Size: 4

Ingredients:
- Black beans: (400 g, about 14 oz) drained and rinsed
- Corn: (200 g, about 7 oz) fresh or frozen
- Peppers: 1 red and 1 yellow, diced
- Onion: 1 large, chopped
- Garlic: 2 cloves, chopped
- Peeled tomatoes: (400 g, about 14 oz) chopped
- Chili powder: 1 tablespoon
- Cumin: 1 teaspoon
- Extra virgin olive oil: 2 tablespoons
- Salt and pepper: to taste
- Fresh coriander: chopped, for garnish
- Avocado: 1, diced, for garnish

Instructions:
Preparation of Sofritto:
- In a large pot, heat extra virgin olive oil over medium heat.
- Add onion and garlic and sauté until transparent.

Adding the Spices and Peppers:

- Incorporate the chili powder and cumin, stirring for about a minute until fragrant.
- Add peppers and cook for another 5 minutes.

Cooking Chili:
- Add peeled tomatoes, black beans, and corn.
- Let simmer for at least 30 minutes, stirring occasionally.
- If the chili appears too thick, add a little water to reach the desired consistency.
- Season with salt and pepper to taste.

Service:
- Serve the chili hot, garnished with fresh chopped cilantro and avocado cubes.

Advice:
- For a spicy touch, add a fresh chopped chili pepper while cooking.
- Serve with a lime wedge to splash some fresh juice before eating.

Eggplant lasagna with ricotta and spinach

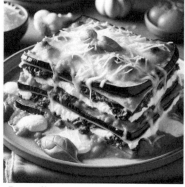

Nutritional Values per Serving:
- Calories: about 350 kcal
- Protein: 18 g
- Fats: 20 g
- Carbohydrates: 25 g
- Fiber: 6 g
- Sugars: 8 g

Preparation Time: 30 minutes
Cooking Time: 30 minutes
Serving Size: 4

Advice:
- For a lighter version, use low-fat cottage cheese and part-skim mozzarella.
- Add fresh basil or oregano for an additional touch of Mediterranean flavor.

Ingredients:
- Eggplant: 2 large, cut into long slices
- Ricotta cheese: 250 g (approximately 8.82 oz)
- Spinach: 300 g (approximately 10.58 oz)
- Tomato puree: 400 ml (approximately 13.53 fl oz or 1.69 cups)
- Mozzarella cheese: 100 g (approximately 3.53 oz)
- Garlic: 2 cloves, chopped
- Extra virgin olive oil: for cooking
- Salt and pepper: to taste
- Nutmeg: a pinch
- Parmesan cheese: for garnish

Instructions:
Preparing Eggplant:
- Brush the eggplant slices with extra virgin olive oil and season with salt and pepper.
- Grill the slices on a grill pan until they are soft and slightly charred, about 2-3 minutes per side.

Preparation of Spinach and Ricotta Stuffing:

- In a bowl, mix ricotta cheese with chopped spinach, garlic, nutmeg, salt and pepper until smooth.

Assembling Lasagna:
- In a baking dish, pour a thin layer of tomato puree.
- Arrange a layer of eggplant slices, then spread some of the ricotta and spinach filling on top.
- Repeat the layers until you run out of ingredients, ending with a final layer of eggplant.
- Sprinkle the surface with grated mozzarella and Parmesan cheese.

Cooking:
- Bake in a preheated 190°C oven for 25-30 minutes, until the surface is golden brown and hot.

Service:
- Let the lasagna rest for 10 minutes before serving to stabilize the layers.

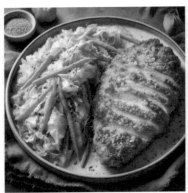

Baked turkey cutlets with oatmeal breadcrumbs

Nutritional Values per Serving:
- Calories: about 350 kcal
- Protein: 30 g
- Fats: 15 g
- Carbohydrates: 20 g
- Fiber: 4 g
- Sugars: 5 g

Preparation Time: 15 minutes
Cooking Time: 25 minutes
Serving Size: 4

Ingredients:
- Turkey breast: 4 slices (about 150 g each) / approximately 5.29 oz each
- Oat flakes: 100 g / approximately 3.53 oz, finely chopped
- Eggs: 2, lightly beaten
- Cabbage: 300 g / approximately 10.58 oz, finely chopped
- Carrots: 2 medium, grated
- Extra virgin olive oil: for seasoning
- Apple vinegar: 2 tablespoons
- Mustard: 1 tablespoon
- Honey: 1 teaspoon
- Salt and pepper: to taste

Instructions:

Preparation of Cutlets:
- Preheat the oven to 200°C.
- Dip the turkey slices first in the beaten egg and then in the chopped oatmeal, making sure they are well covered.
- Place the cutlets on a baking sheet lined with parchment paper and bake for 20 to 25 minutes until golden brown.

Preparation of Kale Salad:
- In a large bowl, mix chopped cabbage and grated carrots.
- In a smaller bowl, combine extra virgin olive oil, apple cider vinegar, mustard, and honey to create the dressing.
- Pour the dressing over the coleslaw and mix well.

Service:
- Serve the turkey cutlets hot accompanied by the fresh coleslaw.

Advice:
- For a gluten-free version, make sure the oatmeal is certified gluten-free.
- Add sunflower or pumpkin seeds to the salad for a crunchy touch.

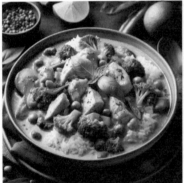

Thai green curry with chicken and vegetables

Nutritional Values per Serving:
- Calories: about 400 kcal
- Protein: 25 g
- Fats: 20 g
- Carbohydrates: 30 g
- Fiber: 3 g
- Sugars: 5 g

Preparation Time: 15 minutes
Cooking Time: 20 minutes
Serving Size: 4

Ingredients:
- Chicken breast: 400 g (14 oz), cut into cubes
- Coconut milk: 400 ml (13.5 fl oz)
- Green curry paste: 2 tablespoons (2 tbsp)
- Broccoli: 100 g (3.5 oz), cut into small florets
- Peppers: 1 green, cut into strips
- Onion: 1 medium, sliced
- Thai basil: a handful, leaves
- Extra virgin olive oil: 1 tablespoon
- Steamed rice: to serve
- Salt and pepper: to taste
- Limes: 1, for garnish
- Fresh coriander: for garnish
- **Instructions:**

Curry Preparation:
- Heat oil in a large frying pan or wok over medium heat.
- Add green curry paste and sauté for one minute to release its flavors.
- Pour in the coconut milk and bring to a gentle boil.

Cooking Chicken and Vegetables:
- Add the chicken to the skillet and cook until almost fully cooked.
- Integrate the broccoli, peppers, and onion, cooking until the vegetables are tender but still crisp.

Final and Service:
- Season with salt and pepper, and add the Thai basil leaves.
- Serve the hot curry over the steamed rice.
- Garnish with lime wedges and chopped fresh cilantro.

Advice:
- Be sure to use a good quality green curry paste for the best flavor.
- Varies vegetables according to season or personal preference.

Brown rice paella with seafood and vegetables

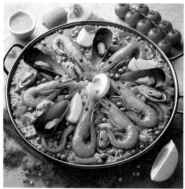

Nutritional Values per Serving:
- Calories: about 450 kcal
- Protein: 25 g
- Fats: 15 g
- Carbohydrates: 55 g
- Fiber: 6 g
- Sugars: 4 g

Preparation Time: 20 minutes
Cooking Time: 40 minutes
Serving Size: 4

Ingredients:
- Brown rice: 300 g (10.6 oz)
- Assorted seafood (shrimp, mussels, squid): 400 g (14 oz)
- Peppers: 1 red and 1 yellow, cut into strips
- Frozen peas: 100 g (3.5 oz)
- Tomatoes: 2 medium, chopped
- Onion: 1 large, chopped
- Garlic: 2 cloves, chopped
- Saffron: 1 sachetFish broth: 800 ml
- Extra virgin olive oil: 3 tablespoons
- Salt and pepper: to taste
- Lemon: 1, cut into wedges for garnish
- Fresh parsley: chopped, for garnish

Instructions:
Preparation of Rice and Seafood:
- Rinse brown rice well under cold running water.
- Clean the seafood, making sure it is free of impurities.

Cooking Paella:

- In a large paellera or large skillet, heat extra virgin olive oil over medium heat.
- Fry the onion and garlic until translucent.
- Add chopped peppers and tomatoes and cook for a few minutes.
- Incorporate the rice and stir well to toast it lightly.
- Add the hot fish stock, peas, and saffron. Bring to a boil, then reduce heat and let cook covered for about 30 minutes.
- Arrange the seafood on top of the rice and cover the pan. Let cook until the seafood is cooked and the rice is tender.

Final and Service:
- Taste and adjust salt and pepper if necessary.
- Serve the paella straight from the pan, garnished with lemon wedges and fresh chopped parsley.

Advice:
- Be sure not to stir the rice once you add the seafood to allow the "socarrat," the crispy crust on the bottom typical of paella, to form.

Buckwheat salad with cherry tomatoes

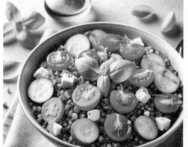

Nutritional Values per Serving:
- Calories: about 300 kcal
- Protein: 10 g
- Fats: 15 g
- Carbohydrates: 35 g
- Fiber: 5 g
- Sugars: 5 g

Preparation Time: 15 minutes
Cooking Time: 0 minutes (if buckwheat is already cooked)
Portions: 4

Ingredients:
- Buckwheat: 200 g (7 oz), cooked
- Cherry tomatoes: 150 g (5.3 oz), cut in half
- Cucumbers: 1 large, diced
- Feta cheese: 100 g (3.5 oz), crumbled
- Extra virgin olive oil: 3 tablespoons (3 tbsp)
- Balsamic vinegar: 1 tablespoon (1 tbsp)
- Salt and pepper: to taste
- Fresh basil: chopped, for garnish

Instructions:
Salad preparation:
- In a large bowl, combine cooked buckwheat, chopped cherry tomatoes, diced cucumbers, and crumbled feta.

Seasoning:
- In a smaller bowl, mix the extra virgin olive oil with the balsamic vinegar.
- Season with salt and pepper to suit your taste.

Assembly and Service:
- Pour the dressing over the buckwheat and vegetable mixture.
- Mix well to ensure that all ingredients are evenly seasoned.
- Garnish with chopped fresh basil before serving.
- lemon juice

Advice:
- For a touch of crunch, add toasted sunflower or pumpkin seeds.
- If you prefer a citrusy touch, replace the balsamic vinegar with.

Chicken souvlaki with Greek yogurt tzatziki and Greek salad

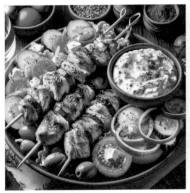

Nutritional Values per Serving:
- Calories: about 450 kcal
- Protein: 35 g
- Fats: 25 g
- Carbohydrates: 20 g
- Fiber: 3 g
- Sugars: 5 g

**Preparation Time: 45 minutes
(plus marinating time)
Cooking Time: 12 minutes
Portions: 4**

Ingredients:
For the Chicken Souvlaki:
- Chicken breast: 400 g, (14 oz) diced
- Extra virgin olive oil: 2 tablespoons
- Lemon juice: 1 lemon
- Garlic: 2 cloves, chopped
- Oregano: 1 teaspoon, dried
- Salt and pepper: to taste

For the Tzatziki:
- Greek yogurt: 200 g (7oz)
- Cucumber: 1 small, grated and drained
- Garlic: 1 clove, chopped
- Extra virgin olive oil: 1 tablespoon
- White wine vinegar: 1 teaspoon
- Salt and pepper: to taste

For the Greek Salad:
- Tomatoes: 2 medium, cut into pieces
- Cucumbers: 1 medium, cut into pieces
- Red onion: ½, thinly sliced
- Kalamata olives: 50 g (1.7 oz)
- Feta cheese: 100 g, (3.5 oz)crumbled
- Extra virgin olive oil: 2 tablespoons
- Red wine vinegar: 1 tablespoon
- Oregano: 1 teaspoon, dried
- Salt and pepper: to taste

Instructions:
Preparation of Chicken Souvlaki:
- In a bowl, mix oil, lemon juice, minced garlic, oregano, salt and pepper.
- Add the chicken cubes and marinate for at least 30 minutes, preferably several hours in the refrigerator.
- Thread the chicken on skewers and grill over medium-high heat until cooked through, about 10-12 minutes, turning frequently.

Tzatziki preparation:
- Mix Greek yogurt with grated cucumber, garlic, extra virgin olive oil, white wine vinegar, salt and pepper.
- Let rest in the refrigerator for at least 30 minutes before serving to let the flavors meld.

Preparation of Greek Salad:
- In a large bowl, combine tomatoes, cucumbers, red onion, olives, and feta.
- Season with extra virgin olive oil, red wine vinegar, oregano, salt and pepper.

Service:
- Serve the chicken souvlaki hot accompanied by the tzatziki and Greek salad.

Advice:
- For a lighter version, use skinless chicken breast and low-fat Greek yogurt.

Beef tagliata with arugula, cherry tomatoes and parmesan shavings

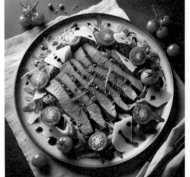

Nutritional Values per Serving:
- Calories: about 400 kcal
- Protein: 32 g
- Fat: 28 g
- Carbohydrates: 4 g
- Fiber: 1 g
- Sugars: 2 g

**Preparation Time: 10 minutes
Cooking Time: 8 minutes
Portions: 2**

Ingredients:
- Beef steak: 400 g (14 oz), preferably sirloin or entrecôte
- Arugula: 100 g (3.5 oz)
- Cherry tomatoes: 150 g (5.3 oz), cut in half
- Parmesan cheese: 50 g (1.8 oz), in flakes
- Extra virgin olive oil: 3 tablespoons (3 tbsp)
- Balsamic vinegar: 1 tablespoon (1 tbsp)
- Salt and black pepper: to taste

Instructions:
Cooking the Steak:
- Season the steak with salt and pepper.
- Heat a frying pan over medium-high heat and add a drizzle of extra virgin olive oil.
- Cook the steak for about 3-4 minutes per side for medium-rare or more depending on preference.
- Let the meat rest for a few minutes before cutting it into thin slices.

Salad preparation:
- In a large bowl, mix the arugula, cherry tomatoes, and parmesan flakes.
- Season with extra virgin olive oil and balsamic vinegar.

Assembly and Service:
- Arrange the warm slices of beef over the bed of arugula, cherry tomatoes, and Parmesan cheese.
- Drizzle with an additional drizzle of oil and a little balsamic vinegar if desired.
- Serve immediately.

Advice:
- For extra flavor, add a pinch of crushed red pepper over the steak before serving.
- A squeeze of fresh lemon on the meat before cutting it can add a hint of freshness.

Lentil burger on a bed of salad with tzatziki sauce

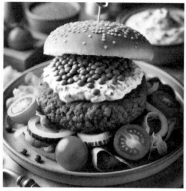

Nutritional Values per Serving:
- Calories: about 350 kcal
- Protein: 18 g
- Fats: 12 g
- Carbohydrates: 42 g
- Fiber: 10 g
- Sugars: 5 g

Preparation Time: 45 minutes (including resting time)
Baking Time: 10 minutes
Portions: 4

Ingredients:
For the Lentil Burger:
- Red lentils: 200 g (7 oz), cooked and mashed
- Onion: 1 small, finely chopped
- Garlic: 1 clove, chopped
- Breadcrumbs: 50 g (1.8 oz)
- Egg: 1 (optional, can be substituted with a vegan binder such as water and flax meal)
- Cumin: 1 teaspoon
- Coriander: 1 teaspoon, ground
- Salt and pepper: to taste
- Extra virgin olive oil: for cooking

For the Tzatziki Sauce:
- Greek yogurt: 150 g (5.3 oz)
- Cucumber: ½, grated and drained
- Garlic: 1 clove, chopped
- Lemon juice: 1 tablespoon (1 tbsp)
- Fresh dill: chopped, to taste
- Salt and pepper: to taste

For the Bed of Salad:
- Green salad mix: 150 g (5.3 oz)
- Cherry tomatoes: 100 g (3.5 oz), cut in half
- Extra virgin olive oil: 1 tablespoon (1 tbsp)
- Balsamic vinegar: 1 teaspoon (1 tsp)

Instructions:
Preparation of Lentil Burgers:
- In a bowl, mix crushed lentils, onion, garlic, breadcrumbs, egg, cumin, coriander, salt and pepper.
- Form burgers from the resulting dough and let them rest in the refrigerator for 30 minutes.
- Cook the burgers in a skillet with extra virgin olive oil until golden brown on both sides.

Preparation of Tzatziki Sauce:
- Combine Greek yogurt, grated cucumber, garlic, lemon juice, dill, salt and pepper in a bowl. Mix well and let stand in refrigerator.

Salad preparation:
- In a bowl, mix green salad mix, cherry tomatoes, extra virgin olive oil and balsamic vinegar.

Assembly and Service:
- Arrange a bed of salad on each plate.
- Place a lentil burger on each bed of salad.
- Add a spoonful of tzatziki sauce on top of each burger.

Advice:
- For a completely vegan version, replace the Greek yogurt with soy yogurt and eliminate the egg, using a vegan substitute to bind the burgers.

Chicken cacciatore with tomatoes, olives and capers

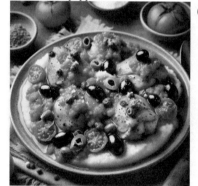

Nutritional Values per Serving:
- Calories: about 550 kcal
- Protein: 35 g
- Fats: 30 g
- Carbohydrates: 35 g
- Fiber: 4 g
- Sugars: 5 g

Preparation Time: 20 minutes
Baking Time: 70 minutes
Portions: 4

Ingredients:
- Chicken thighs: 4
- Peeled tomatoes: 400 g (approximately 14.11 oz), chopped
- Black olives: 100 g (approximately 3.53 oz), pitted
- Capers: 2 tablespoons, rinsed
- Onion: 1 medium, chopped
- Garlic: 2 cloves, chopped
- Red wine: 100 ml (approximately 3.38 fl oz or about 0.42 cups)
- Extra virgin olive oil: 2 tablespoons
- Rosemary: 1 sprig - Salt and pepper: to taste

Ingredients for Soft Polenta:
- Cornmeal for polenta: 200 g (approximately 7.05 oz)
- Water: 1 L (approximately 33.81 fl oz or about 4.23 cups)
- Butter: 30 g (approximately 1.06 oz)
- Parmigiano Reggiano cheese: 50 g (approximately 1.76 oz), grated

Instructions:
Preparation of Chicken Cacciatora:
- In a large skillet, heat extra virgin olive oil and brown the chicken thighs until golden brown on both sides.
- Remove chicken and set aside. In the same pan, add onion and garlic and sauté until transparent.
- Add the peeled tomatoes, olives, capers and rosemary. Pour in the red wine and let it evaporate.
- Return the chicken to the pan, cover, and let it simmer for about 30 minutes.

Preparation of Soft Polenta:
- In a pot, bring salted water to a boil. Slowly pour in the cornmeal, stirring constantly to avoid lumps.
- Reduce the heat and continue cooking, stirring often, until the polenta thickens (about 40 minutes).
- Remove from heat and incorporate butter and Parmesan cheese.

Service:
- Serve the chicken cacciatore hot over a bed of soft polenta, making sure to include plenty of sauce with tomatoes, olives, and capers.

Advice:
- For a richer flavor, you can add a small piece of chopped bacon while sautéing onion and garlic.

Avocado boats with crab and fennel salad

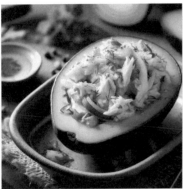

Nutritional Values per Serving:
- Calories: about 300 kcal
- Protein: 10 g
- Fats: 22 g
- Carbohydrates: 12 g
- Fiber: 7 g
- Sugars: 3 g

Preparation Time: 20 minutes
Cooking Time: 0 minutes
Serving Size: 4

Ingredients:
- For Avocado Bars:
- Avocados: 2 large, cut in half and pitted
- Lemon: the juice of 1 lemon
- For the Crab and Fennel Salad:
- Crab meat: 200 g, (7 oz) shelled
- Fennel: 1 bulb, finely chopped
- Red onion: 1 small, finely chopped
- Fresh parsley: chopped, to taste
- Extra virgin olive oil: 2 tablespoons
- Apple vinegar: 1 tablespoon
- Salt and pepper: to taste

Instructions:

Preparation of Avocado Barchettas:
- Sprinkle avocado halves with lemon juice to prevent oxidation.

Preparation of Crab and Fennel Salad:

- In a bowl, mix crab meat, chopped fennel, red onion, parsley, extra virgin olive oil, and apple cider vinegar.
- Season with salt and pepper to taste.

Assembly:
- Fills avocado cavities with crab and fennel salad.

Service:
- Serve the avocado boats immediately to maintain freshness and prevent the avocado from turning brown.

Advice:
- For a spicy note, add a pinch of chili flakes to the crab salad.
- A sprinkling of fennel seeds can add an extra touch of anise flavor to the dish.

Steamed clams with garlic, parsley and a drizzle of extra virgin olive oil

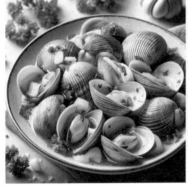

Nutritional Values per Serving:
- Calories: about 200 kcal
- Protein: 15 g
- Fats: 10 g
- Carbohydrates: 5 g
- Fiber: 0 g
- Sugars: 0 g

Preparation Time: 30 minutes (including purification time of clams)
Cooking Time: 10 minutes
Portions: 4

Ingredients:
- Clams: 1 kg (2.2 lbs), well cleaned
- Garlic: 4 cloves, sliced thinly
- Fresh parsley: chopped, to taste
- Extra virgin olive oil: 3 tablespoons (3 tbsp)
- White wine: 100 ml (3.4 fl oz)
- Black pepper: freshly ground, to taste
- **Instructions:**

Preparation of Clams:
- Make sure the clams are clean. Leave them in cold salted water for about 20 minutes, then rinse them under running water to remove any residual sand.

Cooking Clams:
- In a large skillet with a lid, heat extra virgin olive oil over medium heat.
- Add sliced garlic and sauté until golden brown.
- Add the clams and white wine, then cover and let cook for about 5-7 minutes, until all the clams have opened.
- Discard those that did not open.

Final and Service:
- Using a slotted spoon, transfer the clams to serving dishes.
- Strain the liquid remaining in the pan through a fine strainer to remove any residue.
- Drizzle the clams with the strained liquid and a drizzle of extra virgin olive oil.
- Sprinkle with plenty of chopped parsley and a grinding of black pepper.
- Serve immediately.

Advice:
- Serve the clams with slices of toasted crusty bread to soak up the delicious broth.
- For a spicy touch, add a small piece of fresh red pepper along with garlic.

Quinoa salad with avocado, mango and shrimp

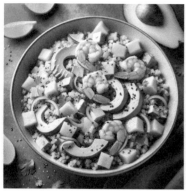

Nutritional Values per Serving:
- Calories: about 350 kcal
- Protein: 15 g
- Fats: 15 g
- Carbohydrates: 40 g
- Fiber: 5 g
- Sugars: 10 g

Preparation Time: 20 minutes
Cooking Time: 15 minutes
Serving Size: 4

Ingredients:
For the Quinoa Salad:
- Quinoa: 200 g (7 oz), cooked
- Avocado: 1 large, diced
- Mango: 1 medium, diced
- Shrimp: 200 g (7 oz), shelled and cooked
- Red onion: 1 small, finely chopped
- Fresh coriander: chopped, to taste
- Lime: the juice of 2 limes
- Extra virgin olive oil: 2 tablespoons (2 tbsp)
- Salt and pepper: to taste

Instructions:
Preparation of Quinoa:
- Rinse the quinoa under cold water and cook it according to package instructions. Let it cool completely.

Preparation of Shrimp:
- Cook the shrimp in a skillet with a drizzle of oil until they are pink and fully cooked. Let them cool.

Salad Assembly:
- In a large bowl, combine cold quinoa, avocado cubes, mango cubes, cooked shrimp, red onion, and fresh cilantro.
- Season with lime juice, extra virgin olive oil, salt and pepper.
- Mix gently to combine all ingredients without crushing the avocado.

Service:
- Serve the salad fresh, ideal as a main course or as a rich and colorful side dish.

Advice:
- For a spicy touch, add a small piece of chopped fresh chili to the salad.
- Be sure to use a ripe mango for natural sweetness and a smooth texture.

Peppers stuffed with quinoa and vegetables

Nutritional Values per Serving:
- Calories: about 250 kcal
- Protein: 9 g
- Fats: 12 g
- Carbohydrates: 28 g
- Fiber: 5 g
- Sugars: 8 g

Preparation Time: 20 minutes
Cooking Time: 40 minutes
Serving Size: 4

Ingredients:
- Peppers: 4 large, cut in half and drained
- Quinoa: 150 g (5.3 oz), cooked
- Zucchini: 1 medium, chopped
- Carrots: 1 large, shredded
- Onion: 1 small, chopped
- Garlic: 2 cloves, chopped
- Peeled tomatoes: 200 g (7 oz), chopped
- Feta cheese: 100 g (3.5 oz), crumbled
- Extra virgin olive oil: 2 tablespoons (2 tbsp)
- Salt and pepper: to taste
- Herbs (basil, parsley): chopped, to taste

Instructions:
Preparation of Quinoa and Vegetables:
- Heat oil in a large skillet over medium heat. Add the onion and garlic and sauté until translucent.
- Add chopped zucchini and carrots; cook until soft.
- Incorporate cooked quinoa and peeled tomatoes; cook for another 5 minutes. Season with salt, pepper and herbs.

Filling the Peppers:
- Preheat the oven to 190°C.
- Fill each bell pepper half with the quinoa and vegetable mixture.
- Sprinkle the surface with crumbled feta cheese.

Baking:
- Arrange the stuffed peppers in a baking dish.
- Cover with aluminum foil and bake in the oven for about 30 minutes.
- Remove the aluminum foil and bake for another 10 minutes or until the peppers are tender and the cheese is golden brown.

Service:
- Serve the peppers hot, garnished with additional fresh herbs if desired.

Advice:
- For a vegan version, replace the feta cheese with a vegan cheese or simply omit it.
- Add chickpeas or black beans to increase the protein content of the filling.

Grilled mackerel with grilled eggplant and mint

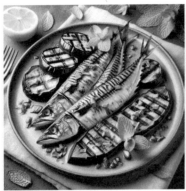

Nutritional Values per Serving:
- Calories: about 350 kcal
- Protein: 25 g
- Fats: 25 g
- Carbohydrates: 5 g
- Fiber: 2 g
- Sugars: 3 g

Preparation Time: 15 minutes
Cooking Time: 10 minutes
Serving Size: 4

Ingredients:
For Grilled Mackerel:
- Mackerel: 4 fillets
- Extra virgin olive oil: for brushing
- Salt and pepper: to taste
- Lemon: 1, cut into wedges for serving

For Grilled Eggplant:
- Eggplant: 2 large, cut into slices 1 cm thick
- Extra virgin olive oil: for brushing
- Salt and pepper: to taste

For Seasoning:
- Fresh mint: chopped, to taste
- Garlic: 1 clove, chopped
- White wine vinegar: 2 tablespoons
- Extra virgin olive oil: 3 tablespoons

Instructions:
Preparation of Mackerel and Eggplant:
- Preheat the grill or a grill on medium-high heat.
- Brush the mackerel fillets and eggplant slices with extra virgin olive oil and season with salt and pepper.
- Grill the mackerel for about 2 to 3 minutes per side, until it is well cooked and the skin is crispy.
- Grill the eggplant slices for about 3-4 minutes per side, until they are tender and marked from the grill.

Preparation of Seasoning:
- In a small bowl, mix chopped fresh mint, garlic, white wine vinegar, and extra virgin olive oil.

Assembly and Service:
- Arrange the grilled eggplant slices on a serving platter.
- Lay the grilled mackerel fillets on top of the eggplant.
- Drizzle mint dressing over mackerel and eggplant.
- Serve with lemon wedges on the side.

Advice:
- Make sure the grill is hot before adding mackerel and eggplant to prevent sticking.
- The mint adds a contrasting freshness that balances well the rich taste of the mackerel.

Grilled tuna steak with avocado and cilantro sauce.

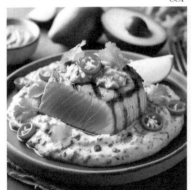

Nutritional Values per Serving:
- Calories: about 350 kcal
- Protein: 25 g
- Fats: 25 g
- Carbohydrates: 5 g
- Fiber: 3 g
- Sugars: 1 g

Preparation Time: 15 minutes
Cooking Time: 5 minutes
Portions: 4

Ingredients:
For Tuna Steak:
- Tuna fillets: 4 (about 200 g, 7 oz each)
- Extra virgin olive oil: for brushing
- Salt and pepper: to taste
- **For the Avocado and Cilantro Sauce:**
- Avocado: 1 large, ripe
- Fresh cilantro: one bunch, chopped
- Lime: the juice of 2 limes
- Red chili pepper: 1, finely chopped (optional)
- Salt and pepper: to taste

Instructions:
Tuna Preparation:
- Preheat the grill to medium-high heat.
- Brush the tuna fillets with extra virgin olive oil and season with salt and pepper.
- Grill the tuna for about 1-2 minutes per side for medium rare, or more depending on personal preference.

Preparation of Avocado and Cilantro Salsa:
- Peel and mash the avocado in a bowl to a creamy consistency.
- Add chopped cilantro, lime juice, chopped chili, salt and pepper.
- Mix well until the ingredients are fully combined.

Service:
- Arrange grilled tuna steaks on plates.
- Accompany each fillet with a generous portion of avocado and cilantro salsa.
- Garnish with lime slices or additional chopped fresh cilantro, if desired.

Advice:
- Be sure not to overcook the tuna to maintain its tender and juicy texture.
- Avocado and cilantro salsa can be prepared in advance and stored in the refrigerator until serving to intensify the flavors.

Turkey meatloaf with spinach and spices

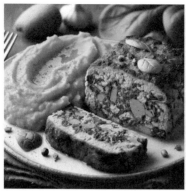

Nutritional Values per Serving:
- Calories: about 450 kcal
- Protein: 35 g
- Fats: 20 g
- Carbohydrates: 35 g
- Fiber: 5 g
- Sugars: 8 g

Preparation Time: 30 minutes
Baking Time: 70 minutes
Portions: 4

Ingredients:
For Turkey Meatloaf:
- Ground turkey: 500 g (17.6 oz)
- Spinach: 200 g (7 oz), chopped and squeezed
- Onion: 1 medium, finely chopped
- Garlic: 2 cloves, chopped
- Egg: 1
- Breadcrumbs: 50 g (1.8 oz)Smoked paprika: 1 teaspoon
- Salt and pepper: to taste
- Extra virgin olive oil: for greasing

For Mashed Sweet Potatoes:
- Sweet potatoes: 600 g (21 oz), peeled and cut into cubes
- Butter: 30 g (1 oz)
- Milk: 100 ml (3.4 fl oz)Salt and pepper: to taste
- Nutmeg: a pinch

Instructions:
Preparation of Meatloaf:
- Preheat the oven to 180°C (350°F).

- In a large bowl, mix ground turkey, spinach, onion, garlic, egg, bread crumbs, smoked paprika, salt and pepper.
- Shape the mixture into a patty and place on a baking sheet lined with baking paper lightly greased with oil.
- Bake for about 40-50 minutes or until the meatloaf is cooked and golden brown.

Preparation of Mashed Sweet Potatoes:
- Put sweet potatoes in a pot and cover with water. Bring to a boil and cook until soft, about 20 minutes.
- Drain the potatoes and mash them with a potato masher or blender.
- Add butter, milk, salt, pepper, and nutmeg. Blend until smooth and creamy puree.

Service:
- Cut the meatloaf into slices and serve hot accompanied by the mashed sweet potatoes.

Advice:
- Add fresh herbs such as parsley or chopped cilantro.

Lemon Rosemary Chicken with Roasted Vegetables

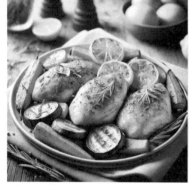

Nutritional Information per Serving:
- Calories: approximately 350 kcal
- Protein: 30 g
- Fat: 15 g
- Carbohydrates: 25 g
- Fiber: 6 g
- Sugars: 5 g

Preparation Time: 15 minutes
Cooking Time: 30 minutes
Servings: 4

Ingredients:
- Chicken breast fillets: 4 (about 150 g / 5.3 oz each)
- Lemon: 1, juice and zest
- Garlic: 2 cloves, minced
- Fresh rosemary: 2 sprigs, chopped
- Sweet potatoes: 2 medium, cubed
- Carrots: 3, sliced
- Zucchini: 2, sliced
- Extra virgin olive oil: 3 tablespoons
- Salt and pepper: to taste
- Fresh parsley: chopped, for garnish

Instructions:
- Marinate the Chicken:
- In a bowl, mix the lemon juice and zest, minced garlic, chopped rosemary, 1 tablespoon of extra virgin olive oil, salt, and pepper.
- Add the chicken fillets to the marinade and mix well. Cover and refrigerate for at least 30 minutes.
- Prepare the Vegetables:
- Preheat the oven to 200°C (392°F).
- In a large baking dish, arrange the sweet potatoes, carrots, and zucchini. Drizzle with 2 tablespoons of extra virgin olive oil, and season with salt and pepper. Toss well to coat evenly.

Cooking:
- Roast the vegetables in the oven for 20 minutes.
- Meanwhile, heat a non-stick skillet over medium-high heat. Remove the chicken from the marinade and cook the fillets for about 4-5 minutes per side, until golden brown and cooked through.
- After 20 minutes, add the chicken to the baking dish with the vegetables and continue roasting for another 10 minutes, until the vegetables are tender and the chicken is fully cooked.

Serve:
- Serve the lemon rosemary chicken with the roasted vegetables on a serving platter.
- Garnish with chopped fresh parsley before serving.

Tips:
- You can add other vegetables like bell peppers, red onions, or broccoli for variety.
- For even more flavor, marinate the chicken overnight in the refrigerator.

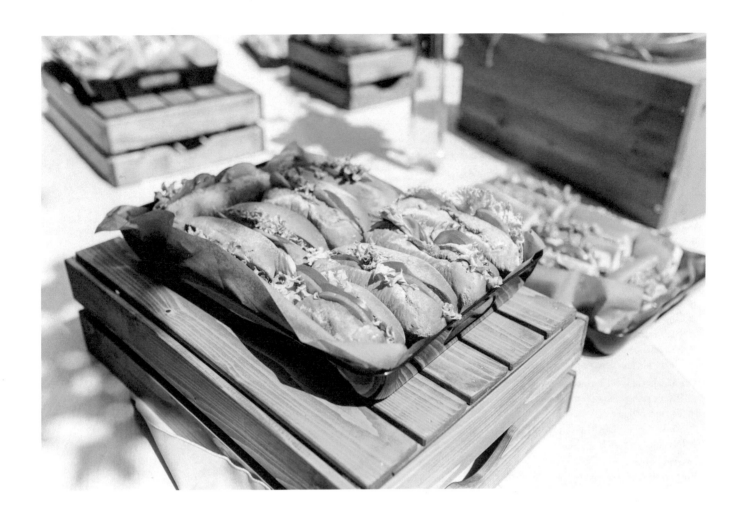

CHAPTER 10: THE HEALTHY AND FLAVORFUL SNACKS.

10.1 Small Delights for Everyday Wellness.

Snacks are a crucial part of a balanced diet, especially for those seeking to maintain or improve liver health. They serve to stabilize blood sugar levels between main meals, preventing spikes and dips that can lead to fatigue and irritability.

In addition, a healthy snack provides sustained energy and helps control appetite, reducing the risk of excesses during meals. Our options are rich in essential nutrients, low in sugar and unhealthy fats, and ideal for supporting a healthy liver and an energetic body.

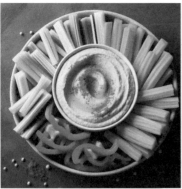

Chickpea Hummus and Crispy Vegetables

Nutritional Values per Serving:
- Calories: about 200 kcal
- Protein: 6 g
- Fats: 10 g
- Carbohydrates: 25 g
- Fiber: 6 g
- Sugars: 5 g

Preparation Time: 10 minutes
Cooking Time: 0 minutes
Portions: 1

Ingredients:
For Hummus:
- Canned chickpeas: (100 g, 3.4 oz) drained and rinsed
- Tahini (sesame paste): 1 tablespoon
- Lemon juice: 1 tablespoon
- Garlic: 1 clove, chopped
- Extra virgin olive oil: 1 teaspoon
- Salt: a pinch
- Paprika: for garnish (optional)
- **For Crispy Vegetables:**
- Carrots: 1 medium, peeled and cut into sticks
- Celery: 1 stalk, cut into sticks
- Red peppers: ¼ bell pepper, cut into sticks

Instructions:
Preparation of Hummus:
- In a blender or food processor, combine the chickpeas, tahini, lemon juice, garlic, extra virgin olive oil, and a pinch of salt.
- Blend until smooth and homogeneous. If necessary, add a

little water to reach the desired consistency.

Service:
- Transfer the hummus to a small bowl and sprinkle with a little paprika for a touch of color and flavor, if desired.
- Arrange the carrot, celery, and bell pepper sticks around the hummus in a serving dish.

Advice:
- Hummus can be stored in the refrigerator in an airtight container for up to a week.
- Vary the vegetables according to preference or seasonality to keep the snack always interesting.

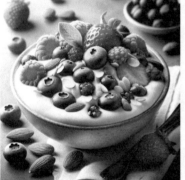

Greek yogurt with berries and almonds

Nutritional Values per Serving:
- Calories: about 180 kcal
- Protein: 10 g
- Fats: 9 g
- Carbohydrates: 18 g
- Fiber: 4 g
- Sugars: 12 g

Preparation Time: 5 minutes
Cooking Time: 0 minutes
Portions: 1

Ingredients:
For Greek Yogurt with Berries and Almonds:
- Greek yogurt: 150 g (5.3 oz), unsweetened
- Blueberries: 50 g (1.8 oz)
- Raspberries: 50 g (1.8 oz)
- Strawberries: 50 g (1.8 oz), cut in halves or quarters depending on size
- Almonds: 15 g (0.5 oz), chopped

Instructions:
Preparation of Yogurt with Berries:
- In a bowl, pour the Greek yogurt.
- Add the blueberries, raspberries, and strawberries on top of the yogurt.

Addition of the Almonds:
- Sprinkle chopped almonds over the berries.

Service:
- Serve immediately to enjoy the freshness of the berries and

the crunchiness of the almonds.

Advice:
- For a variation, you can add a teaspoon of honey or maple syrup if you prefer a natural sweetener.
- Varies berries according to seasonality to diversify flavors and nutritional benefits.

Avocado Stuffed with Tuna

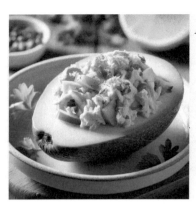

Nutritional Values per Serving:
- Calories: about 300 kcal
- Protein: 15 g
- Fats: 22 g
- Carbohydrates: 9 g
- Fiber: 7 g
- Sugars: 1 g

Preparation Time: 10 minutes
Cooking Time: 0 minutes
Portions: 1

Ingredients:
- For the Avocado Stuffed with Tuna:
- Avocado: 1 large, cut in half and pitted
- Canned natural tuna: 80 g (2.8 oz), drained
- Red onion: 1 small, finely chopped
- Lemon juice: 1 tablespoon
- Salt and pepper: to taste
- Fresh parsley: chopped, for garnish

Instructions:
Preparing Tuna Stuffing:
- In a bowl, mix drained tuna, chopped red onion, lemon juice, salt and pepper until smooth.

Avocado Filling:
- Arrange the avocado halves on a plate.
- Fills each half with the prepared tuna filling.

Service:
- Garnish with fresh chopped parsley before serving.
- Offer as a healthy snack or light appetizer.

Advice:
- For a spicy touch, add a pinch of chili powder or a few drops of hot sauce to the tuna filling.
- Be sure to use a ripe avocado for best texture and flavor.

Mozzarella and Cherry Tomato Skewers

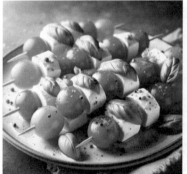

Nutritional Values per Serving:
- Calories: about 150 kcal
- Protein: 8 g
- Fats: 11 g
- Carbohydrates: 5 g
- Fiber: 1 g
- Sugars: 4 g

Preparation Time: 10 minutes
Cooking Time: 0 minutes
Portions: 1-2 (depends on size of skewers)

Ingredients:
- For Mozzarella and Tomato Skewers:
- Mozzarella cheese: 100 g (3.5 oz), preferably low-fat, cut into cubes
- Tomatoes: 8-10, washed
- Fresh basil: 8-10 leaves
- Extra virgin olive oil: 1 tablespoon
- Balsamic vinegar: 1 teaspoon
- Salt and pepper: to taste

Instructions:
Preparing Skewers:
- Thread alternately a mozzarella cube, a basil leaf and a cherry tomato onto toothpicks or small wooden skewers.

Seasoning:
- In a small bowl, mix extra virgin olive oil, balsamic vinegar, salt and pepper.
- Gently brush the seasoning onto the prepared skewers.

Service:
- Arrange the skewers on a serving platter.
- You can serve the skewers immediately or let them marinate for about 10 to 15 minutes in the refrigerator to intensify the flavors.

Advice:
- For an extra touch of flavor, add a pinch of dried oregano or chili flakes to the dressing.
- These skewers are perfect as a light appetizer or as part of an assortment of appetizers.

Spinach and Green Apple Smoothie

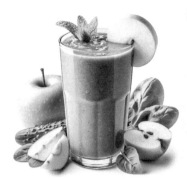

Nutritional Values per Serving:
- Calories: about 120 kcal
- Protein: 2 g
- Fats: 0.5 g
- Carbohydrates: 28 g
- Fiber: 5 g
- Sugars: 20 g

Preparation Time: 5 minutes
Cooking Time: 0 minutes S
ervings: 1

Ingredients:
- For Spinach and Green Apple Smoothie:
- Fresh spinach: 1 cup, well washed
- Green apple: 1, cut into pieces and seedless
- Cucumber: ½, cut into pieces
- Coconut water: 200 ml (6.8 fl oz)
- Lemon juice: 1 tablespoon
- Fresh mint: a few leaves (optional for a touch of freshness)

Instructions:
Smoothie Preparation:
- In a blender, add spinach, green apple, cucumber, coconut water, lemon juice and mint leaves.
- Blend at high speed until smooth and homogeneous.

Service:
- Pour the smoothie into a tall glass.
- If desired, decorate with a slice of green apple or a mint leaf.

Advice:
- You can add a teaspoon of chia or flax seeds to increase the fiber and omega-3 content.
- For a sweeter smoothie, add a little honey or maple syrup to taste.

Whole grain crackers with Guacamole sauce

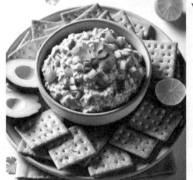

Nutritional Values per Serving:
- Calories: about 200 kcal
- Protein: 3 g
- Fats: 15 g
- Carbohydrates: 18 g
- Fiber: 5 g
- Sugars: 2 g

Preparation Time: 10 minutes
Cooking Time: 0 minutes
Portions: 1-2

Ingredients:
- For Whole Wheat Crackers with Guacamole Sauce:
- Guacamole:
- Avocado: 1 large, ripe
- Lime juice: 1 tablespoon
- Red onion: 2 tablespoons, finely chopped
- Tomatoes: 1 small, chopped
- Fresh coriander: 1 tablespoon, chopped
- Salt and pepper: to taste
- Whole wheat crackers: 8-10 pieces

Instructions:
Preparation of Guacamole:
- Cut the avocado in half, remove the pit and scoop out the pulp with a spoon.
- In a bowl, mash the avocado with a fork until creamy.
- Add lime juice, red onion, chopped tomato, cilantro, salt and pepper.
- Mix all ingredients well until a smooth sauce is obtained.

Service:
- Arrange the whole-grain crackers on a plate.
- Serve the guacamole in a separate bowl or spread it directly on crackers before serving.

Advice:
- Add a pinch of chili powder to guacamole for a spicy touch.
- Be sure to use well-ripened avocados for best creaminess.

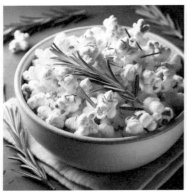

Rosemary Popcorn

Nutritional Values per Serving:
- Calories: about 100 kcal
- Protein: 2 g
- Fat: 6 g
- Carbohydrates: 10 g
- Fiber: 2 g
- Sugars: 0 g

Preparation Time: 5 minutes
Cooking Time: 5 minutes
Portions: 2

Ingredients:
- For Rosemary Popcorn:
- Corn kernels for popcorn: 50 g (1.8 oz)
- Extra virgin olive oil: 1 tablespoon
- Fresh rosemary: 1 sprig, finely chopped
- Sea salt: to taste

Instructions:
Popcorn preparation:
- In a large pot with a lid, heat extra virgin olive oil over medium heat.
- Add the corn kernels and chopped rosemary, stirring to cover the kernels evenly with the oil and rosemary.
- Cover the pot and, once the kernels begin to pop, shake the pot occasionally to prevent the popcorn from burning.
- When the sound of bangs dies down, put out the fire.

Seasoning and Service:
- Sprinkle the hot popcorn with a pinch of sea salt and mix well.
- Serve the popcorn while it is still hot to best enjoy its flavor and crunchiness.

Advice:
- For an oil-free alternative, you can make popcorn in a fat-free popcorn machine.
- For variation, try adding other herbs such as thyme or sage for a different flavor profile.

Cucumbers Stuffed with Ricotta and Herbs

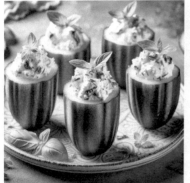

Nutrition Values per Serving:
- Calories: about 50 kcal
- Protein: 3 g
- Fats: 3 g
- Carbohydrates: 2 g
- Fiber: 1 g
- Sugars: 1 g

Preparation Time: 15 minutes
Cooking Time: 0 minutes
Portions: 4 (about 2 cylinders per person)

Ingredients:
- For Cucumbers Stuffed with Ricotta and Herbs:
- Cucumbers: 2 large ones, cut into cylinders of about 2 inches
- Ricotta cheese: 100 g (3.5 oz)
- Fresh herbs (parsley, basil, mint): 2 tablespoons, finely chopped
- Lemon: the zest of 1 lemon
- Salt and pepper: to taste

Instructions:
Preparing Cucumbers:
- Cut the cucumbers into cylinders, then use a teaspoon or sander to remove the center, creating a cavity.

Preparing the Stuffing:
- In a bowl, mix the cottage cheese with the chopped herbs, lemon zest, salt and pepper until smooth.

Filling the Cucumbers:
- Use a teaspoon to fill the cavities of the cucumbers with the cottage cheese and herb mixture.

Service:
- Arrange the stuffed cucumbers on a serving platter.
- You can serve them immediately or let them chill in the refrigerator for an hour before serving to intensify the flavors.

Advice:
- You can vary the herbs according to availability or your preferences to diversify the taste.
- Add a little garlic powder or chopped onion to the filling for a stronger flavor.

Apple Rings with Peanut Butter and Granola

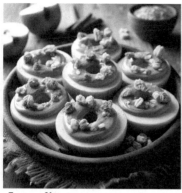

Nutritional Values per Serving:
- Calories: about 200 kcal (depends on the size of the apples and the amount of peanut butter)
- Protein: 4 g
- Fats: 8 g
- Carbohydrates: 30 g
- Fiber: 5 g
- Sugars: 20 g

Preparation Time: 10 minutes
Cooking Time: 0 minutes
Portions: 2-4

Ingredients:
- For Apple Rings with Peanut Butter and Granola:
- Apples: 2 large ones, preferably crisp varieties such as Fuji or Honeycrisp
- Peanut butter: 4 tablespoons, natural and no added sugar
- Granola: 2 tablespoons, no added sugar
- Cinnamon: a pinch for sprinkling (optional)

Instructions:
Preparation of Apples:
- Wash the apples and remove the core. Cut the apples into rings about 1 cm thick.

Assembly:
- Spread one side of each apple ring with peanut butter.
- Sprinkle the granola over the peanut butter and add a pinch of cinnamon, if desired.

Service:
- Arrange the apple rings on a serving platter and serve immediately to retain the crispness of the apples and the freshness of the peanut butter.

Advice:
- Be sure to choose a natural peanut butter with no added sugars to keep the snack as healthy as possible.
- By varying the granola or adding other types of seeds, such as chia seeds or flax seeds, you can add additional nutrients and variety to this snack.

Chicken and Avocado Mini Sandwich

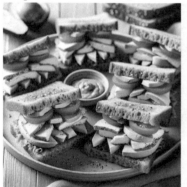

Nutritional Values per Serving:
- Calories: about 250 kcal
- Protein: 15 g
- Fats: 12 g
- Carbohydrates: 20 g
- Fiber: 5 g
- Sugars: 3 g

Preparation Time: 15 minutes
Cooking Time: 0 minutes (assuming the chicken is already cooked)
Portions: 2 (2 mini sandwiches each)

Ingredients:
- For Chicken and Avocado Mini Sandwiches:
- Whole wheat bread: 4 slices, toasted
- Chicken breast: 100 g, (3.5 oz) cooked and sliced
- Avocado: 1 small, ripe, sliced
- Mustard: 2 teaspoons, or to taste
- Lettuce: a few leaves, washed and dried
- Tomatoes: 1 small, sliced
- Salt and pepper: to taste

Instructions:
Preparation of Mini Sandwiches:
- Spread a light amount of mustard on two slices of bread.
- On the first slice, arrange a lettuce leaf, followed by a slice of chicken, a few slices of avocado and tomato.
- Season with salt and pepper to taste.
- Cover with the second slice of bread. Repeat for the second sandwich.

Service:
- Cut sandwiches in half or quarters to create easy-to-eat mini sandwiches.
- Arrange them on a serving plate and serve immediately to maintain freshness.

Advice:
- For a richer variation, add slices of crispy bacon or replace mustard with hummus for a creamier version.
- Mini sandwiches are great for a quick lunch, a picnic, or as part of a buffet.

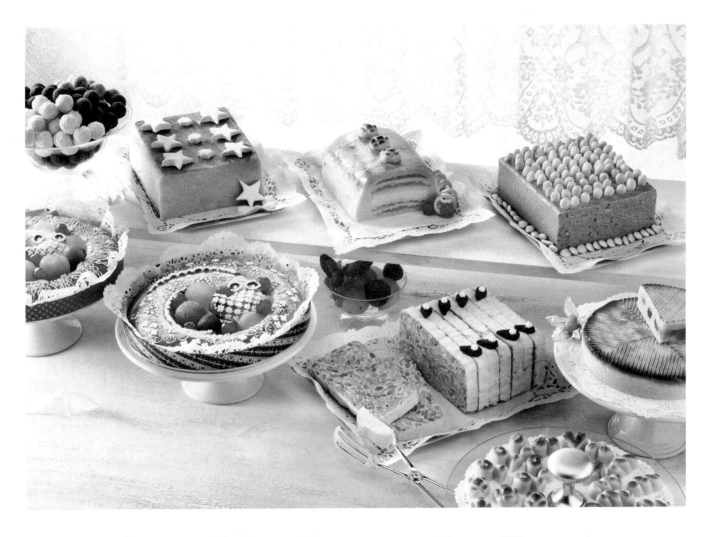

CHAPTER 11: SWEET DELIGHTS FOR LIVER WELLNESS

11.1 The Art of Healthy Desserts

In this chapter, we explore the world of desserts from an extraordinary angle: that of liver health. Who said desserts cannot be part of a balanced diet that benefits our bodies? With a focus on nutritious ingredients and mindful preparation techniques, the desserts presented here are delicious and designed to support liver wellness and keep the body healthy.

Each recipe, from rich and creamy mousses to crunchy cookies, has been carefully developed to minimize added sugars and maximize nutritional benefits. Ingredients such as antioxidant-rich dark chocolate, fresh fruit, and healthy fats have been used. These desserts prove that indulging on a whim without compromising health is possible.

Get ready to delight your palate with these sweets, which will not only put a smile on your face but also contribute to your long-term health. Make room for guilt-free sweetness with these creations designed for pleasure and well-being.

Dark Chocolate and Avocado Mousse

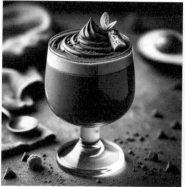

Nutritional Values per Serving:
- Calories: about 350 kcal
- Protein: 4 g
- Fats: 25 g
- Carbohydrates: 30 g
- Fiber: 7 g
- Sugars: 12 g

Preparation Time: 20 minutes
Resting Time: 1 hour
Portions: 4

Ingredients:
- Ripe avocados: 2 large
- 70% dark chocolate: 200 g (7 oz)
- Vanilla essence: 1 teaspoon
- Honey or agave syrup: 3 tablespoons
- Cocoa powder: 2 tablespoons (for dusting)

Instructions:

Chocolate preparation:
- Melt the dark chocolate in a double boiler or in the microwave, being careful not to overheat it.

Preparation of the mousse:
- In a blender, combine the avocado pulp, melted chocolate, vanilla, and honey or agave syrup.
- Blend until smooth and homogeneous.

Rest:
- Pour the mousse into individual cups and let it chill in the refrigerator for at least 1 hour to set.

Finish:
- Before serving, dust with cocoa powder.

Advice:
- For a richer texture, add a pinch of sea salt to the mousse before blending.
- Decorate with berries or a sprinkling of dark chocolate chips for an elegant finishing touch.

Health Benefits:
- This dessert is packed with healthy fats from avocado and antioxidants from dark chocolate.

Presentation:
- Serve the mousse in elegant glass cups, garnished with a sprinkling of cocoa and, if desired, fresh berries or chocolate chips.

Cereal Bars with Dark Chocolate and Red Fruits

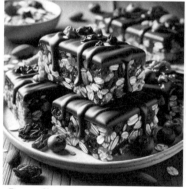

Nutritional Values per Bar:
- Calories: about 220 kcal
- Protein: 4 g
- Fats: 12 g
- Carbohydrates: 25 g
- Fiber: 3 g
- Sugars: 12 g

Preparation Time: 20 minutes
Cooling Time: 30 minutes
Portions: 12 bars

Ingredients:
- Oats: 200 g (7oz)
- Chopped walnuts: 100 g (3.5 oz)
- Honey: 3 tablespoons
- 70% dark chocolate: 100 g, (3.5 oz) chopped
- Dried red fruit mix (blueberries, raspberries, strawberries): 100 g (3.5 oz)
- Coconut butter: 2 tablespoons

Instructions:

Base preparation:
- In a large bowl, mix oats, chopped nuts, and dried red fruits.
- Melt the coconut butter and honey in a small saucepan over low heat, then pour over the oat mixture and stir well.

Bar formation:
- Line a baking sheet with baking paper and pour the mixture on top, pressing well to form an even layer.
- Let cool in the refrigerator for at least 30 minutes.

Adding chocolate:
- Melt the dark chocolate in a double boiler or microwave and pour it evenly over the cooled cereal layer.
- Let the chocolate solidify completely.

Cutting the bars:
- Once the chocolate has solidified, cut the mixture into equal-sized bars.

Advice:
- Store the bars in an airtight container in the refrigerator to maintain freshness.
- You can vary the types of red fruits or nuts according to your preference or availability.

Presentation:
- Serve the bars on a decorative plate, perhaps with some fresh fruit alongside for a colorful touch.

Lemon Ginger Sorbet

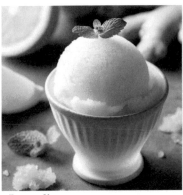

Nutritional Values per Serving:
- Calories: about 70 kcal
- Protein: 1 g
- Fats: 0 g
- Carbohydrates: 18 g
- Fiber: 0 g
- Sugars: 4 g (natural from lemon)

Preparation Time: 20 minutes
Freezing Time: 2-4 hours
Portions: 4

Ingredients:
- Lemons: 4 large, squeezed
- Fresh ginger: 2 cm, (0.79 in)grated
- Water: 500 ml (16.9 fl oz)
- Stevia: 3 tablespoons (or to taste, for sweetening)

Instructions:
Syrup preparation:
- In a small saucepan, bring water with grated ginger and stevia to a boil.
- Reduce the heat and simmer for 5 minutes to allow the ginger to infuse well. Then, let it cool completely.

Mix the ingredients together:
- Strain the syrup to remove the ginger pieces and mix it with fresh lemon juice.

Freeze:
- Pour the mix into an ice cream maker and follow the device's instructions for making sorbet. If you do not have an ice cream maker, pour the mix into a container and place it in the freezer. Stir every hour for the first 4 hours to help break up the ice crystals.

Serve:
- • Serve the sorbet in dessert cups or as balls in waffle cones.

Advice:
- Add a mint leaf or lemon slice for garnish and add a touch of freshness.
- The sorbet is best when eaten the same day, but it can be stored in the freezer for up to a week.

Presentation:
- Serve the sorbet in elegant glass cups, garnished with a slice of lemon or candied ginger for a refined visual effect.

Coconut Mango Panna Cotta

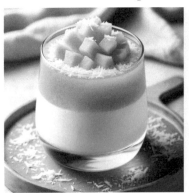

Nutritional Values per Serving:
- Calories: about 280 kcal
- Protein: 2 g
- Fats: 24 g
- Carbohydrates: 15 g
- Fiber: 2 g
- Sugars: 10 g

Preparation Time: 15 minutes
Cooling Time: 4 hours
Portions: 4

Ingredients:
- Coconut milk: 400 ml (13.5 fl)Agar-agar: 2 teaspoons
- Fresh mango pulp: 200 g (7 oz)
- Honey: 2 tablespoons (optional, for sweetening)
- Vanilla extract: 1 teaspoon
- Grated coconut: for garnish

Instructions:
Base preparation:
- In a saucepan, bring the coconut milk with the agar-agar to a boil, stirring constantly until it is completely dissolved.
- Add the honey and vanilla extract, mix well, and cook for another 2 minutes.

Cooling:
- Pour the mixture into dessert cups and let cool to room temperature, then transfer to the refrigerator for at least 4 hours, until solidified.

Preparation of mango topping:
- Blend the mango pulp until smoothly pureed.
- Store the puree in the refrigerator until ready to serve.

Serve:
- When ready to serve, pour mango puree over each panna cotta.
- Garnish with grated coconut.

Advice:
- Make sure the mango is ripe for a sweeter flavor and creamy texture.
- For a more exotic variation, add a pinch of cardamom or turmeric to the mango puree.

Presentation:
- Serve the panna cotta in clear cups to show layers of coconut cream and mango puree, making the dessert visually appealing and inviting.

Walnut Tart with Dark Chocolate

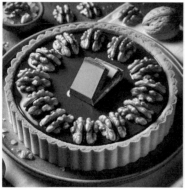

Nutritional Values per Serving:
- Calories: about 320 kcal
- Protein: 6 g
- Fat: 28 g
- Carbohydrates: 12 g
- Fiber: 3 g
- Sugars: 4 g

Preparation Time: 30 minutes
Cooking Time: 25 minutes
Portions: 8

Ingredients:
- Almond flour: 200 g (7 oz)
- Chopped walnuts: 100 g (3.5 oz)
- Butter: 100 g, at room temperature (3.5 oz)
- 70% dark chocolate: 150 g (5.3 oz)
- Eggs: 2 large
- Erythritol: 50 g (1.8 oz) (or other low-sugar sweetener)

Instructions:
Base preparation:
- In a bowl, mix almond flour with chopped walnuts.
- Add the butter and erythritol, working the mixture to a sandy consistency.
- Add one egg at a time, mixing well until a smooth dough is formed.
- Press the dough into a previously buttered tart mold, forming a raised rim on the sides.

Baking the base:
- Preheat the oven to 180°C (350°F) and bake the tart base for 15 minutes, or until lightly browned.

Chocolate preparation:
- Meanwhile, melt the dark chocolate in a double boiler or in the microwave, making sure not to burn it.

Assembly and final firing:
- Pour the melted chocolate over the pre-cooked tart base.
- Return the tart to the oven and bake for another 10 minutes.

Cooling and service:
- Let the tart cool completely before removing it from the mold.
- Cut into portions and serve.

Advice:
- For an extra crispy tart, you can toast the walnuts before chopping them.
- Add a pinch of salt to the melted chocolate to enhance the flavor.

Presentation:
- Serve the tart on a serving platter, garnished with some whipped cream or vanilla ice cream if desired.

Banana and Peanut Butter Ice Cream

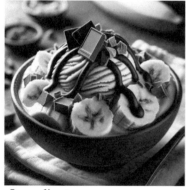

Nutritional Values per Serving:
- Calories: about 280 kcal
- Protein: 6 g
- Fats: 15 g
- Carbohydrates: 30 g
- Fiber: 4 g
- Sugars: 18 g (natural from bananas and peanut butter)

Preparation Time: 10 minutes
Freezing Time: 1-2 hours (optional)
Portions: 4

Ingredients:
- Ripe bananas: 4, frozen and cut into pieces
- Natural peanut butter: 4 tablespoons
- Cocoa powder: 2 tablespoons
- Almond milk: 100 ml (3.4 fl) (adjust according to desired consistency)
- 70% dark chocolate: 50 g, (1.8 oz) chopped for garnish

Instructions:
Ice cream preparation:
- In a high-powered blender, combine the frozen bananas, peanut butter, and cocoa powder.
- Blend at high speed, gradually adding the almond milk until a creamy, smooth ice cream-like consistency is achieved.

Service:
- Serve immediately for a soft ice cream-like consistency or transfer the mixture to a container and freeze for 1-2 hours for a firmer consistency.
- Garnish with chopped dark chocolate before serving.

Advice:
- For an extra touch of flavor, add a sprinkle of sea salt over the ice cream before serving to enhance the flavors.
- Peanut butter can be substituted with another type of nut butter according to preference.

Presentation:
- Serve the ice cream in dessert cups or waffle cones, garnished with chopped dark chocolate for a contrast of texture and flavor.

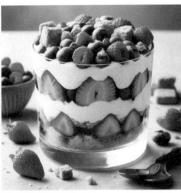

Greek Yogurt and Berry Trifle

Nutritional Values per Serving:
- Calories: about 250 kcal
- Protein: 10 g
- Fats: 6 g
- Carbohydrates: 40 g
- Fiber: 4 g
- Sugars: 28 g

Preparation Time: 15 minutes
Cooling Time: 30 minutes
Portions: 4

Ingredients:
- Greek yogurt: 500 g (17.6. oz)
- Honey: 3 tablespoons
- Vanilla extract: 1 teaspoon
- Mixed fresh berries (strawberries, blueberries, raspberries): 300 g (10.6 oz)
- Crumbled whole wheat cookies: 100 g (3.5 oz)

Instructions:
Yogurt preparation:
- In a bowl, mix Greek yogurt with honey and vanilla extract until smooth.

Trifle assembly:
- In clear dessert cups, start with a layer of crumbled cookies.
- Add a layer of sweetened Greek yogurt.
- Complete with a generous layer of fresh berries.
- Repeat the layers until the cups are filled.

Cooling:
- Let the trifles rest in the refrigerator for at least 30 minutes before serving to allow the flavors to meld.

Advice:
- You can alternate the types of berries to vary the color and taste of the trifle.
- For added crunch, lightly toast the crumbled cookies before adding them to the trifle.

Presentation:
- Serve the trifles in clear glasses to show off the various colored layers, making the dessert not only delicious but also aesthetically pleasing.

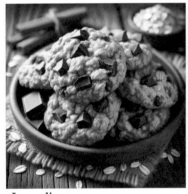

Oatmeal and Dark Chocolate Cookies

Nutritional Values per Biscuit:
- Calories: about 120 kcal
- Protein: 3 g
- Fats: 5 g
- Carbohydrates: 15 g
- Fiber: 2 g
- Sugars: 5 g

Preparation Time: 20 minutes
Baking Time: 15 minutes
Portions: 16 cookies

Ingredients:
- Oat flakes: 200 g (7 oz)
- 70% dark chocolate: 100 g, (3.5oz) chopped
- Ripe banana: 2, mashed
- Eggs: 1 large
- Vanilla extract: 1 teaspoon
- Cinnamon: 1 teaspoon
- Salt: a pinch

Instructions:
Dough preparation:
- In a large bowl, mix oatmeal, chopped dark chocolate, mashed banana, egg, vanilla extract, cinnamon, and salt.
- Make sure all the ingredients are well mixed.

Cookie formation:
- Preheat the oven to 180°C (350°F).
- Line a baking sheet with baking paper.
- With damp hands, form balls of dough and flatten them slightly on the baking sheet, shaping them into cookies.

Cooking:
- Bake the cookies in the oven for 12 to 15 minutes or until golden brown and crispy on the edges.
- Let the cookies cool on the baking sheet for a few minutes before transferring them to a wire rack to complete cooling.

Advice:
- Add chopped nuts or chia seeds for an extra dose of protein and omega-3s.
- The cookies can be stored in an airtight container for up to a week.

Presentation:
- Serve the cookies on a serving platter or in a basket, accompanied by a cup of tea or coffee for a healthy snack.

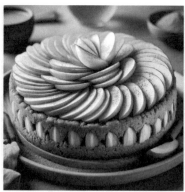

Sugar Free Apple Pie

Nutritional Values per Serving:
- Calories: about 270 kcal
- Protein: 6 g
- Fats: 14 g
- Carbohydrates: 30 g
- Fiber: 4 g
- Sugars: 10 g (natural from apples)

Preparation Time: 20 minutes
Cooking Time: 45 minutes
Portions: 8

Ingredients:
- Apples: 4 large, peeled, cored and sliced
- Whole wheat flour: 200 g (7 oz)
- Eggs: 3 large
- Butter: 100 g, (3.5 oz) at room temperature
- Vanilla extract: 1 teaspoon
- Cinnamon powder: 2 teaspoons
- Baking powder: 1 teaspoon
- Erythritol: 50 g (1.8 oz) (or other natural sweetener of your choice)

Instructions:

Preparation of apples:
- In a bowl, mix apple slices with cinnamon and half the sweetener. Let marinate for about 10 minutes.

Dough preparation:
- In another large bowl, beat the eggs with the remaining sweetener and vanilla extract until frothy.
- Add the soft butter and continue beating.
- Gradually incorporate the flour and baking powder, mixing until the mixture is smooth.

Cake assembly:
- Grease and flour a round cake pan.
- Pour half the batter into the baking dish, then arrange a layer of marinated apples on top.
- Cover with the remaining dough and finish with another layer of apples.

Cooking:
- Bake in a preheated oven at 180°C (350°F) for about 45 minutes or until a toothpick inserted in the center of the cake comes out clean.

Cooling and service:
- Let the cake cool in the pan for 10 minutes, then transfer it to a wire rack to complete cooling.
- Serve the cake possibly warm or at room temperature.

Advice:
- For a spicier variation, add a pinch of ground nutmeg or cloves.
- This cake can be stored in the refrigerator for up to 3 days.

Presentation:
- Serve the cake on a serving platter, garnished with a sprinkle of cinnamon or accompanied by a scoop of vanilla ice cream if desired.

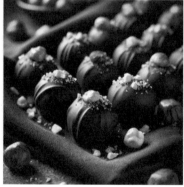

Dark Chocolates Filled with Hazelnuts

Nutritional Values per Chocolate:
- Calories: about 80 kcal
- Protein: 1 g
- Fat: 6 g
- Carbohydrates: 6 g
- Fiber: 1 g
- Sugars: 4 g

Preparation Time: 20 minutes
Cooling Time: 1 hour
Portions: 24 chocolates

Ingredients:
- 70% dark chocolate: 300 g (10.6 oz)
- Roasted hazelnuts: 100 g, (3.7 oz) coarsely chopped
- Sea salt: a pinch

Instructions:

Chocolate preparation:
- Break the dark chocolate into small pieces and melt it in a double boiler or microwave, being careful not to overheat it.

Preparation of chocolates:
- Use chocolate molds or small paper ramekins.
- Pour some melted chocolate into the mold to form the base of the chocolates.
- Add a few chopped hazelnuts to each chocolate base and a pinch of sea salt.
- Top with more melted chocolate until the molds are filled.

Cooling:
- Let the chocolates cool to room temperature for a few minutes, then transfer them to the refrigerator to solidify completely, about 1 hour.

Unmolding and serving:
- Once solidified, remove the chocolates from the molds.
- Serve the chocolates at room temperature for the best balance of texture and flavor.

Advice:
- Make sure the chocolate is of high quality for a better end result.
- Vary the filling by using other types of nuts or adding a touch of cinnamon or chili for different flavors.

Presentation:
- Present the chocolates in an elegant dessert plate or gift box if intended as a sweet gift.

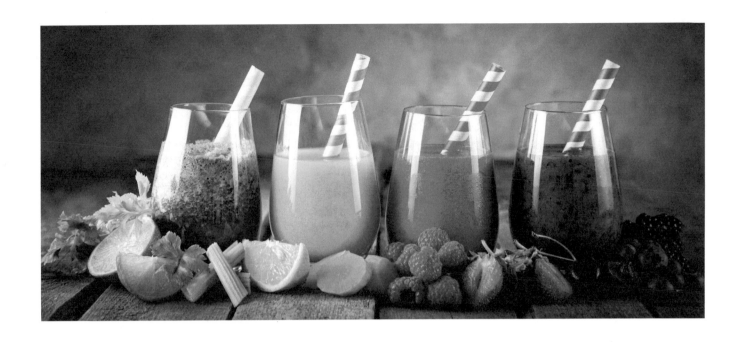

CHAPTER 12: DETOX BEVERAGES FOR LIVER WELLNESS

12.1 The Role of Detox Beverages.

Keeping the liver healthy is critical to overall well-being, and proper hydration is crucial. Drinking beneficial detox liquids helps cleanse the liver, facilitating toxin removal and improving liver function. These drinks support detoxification and provide essential antioxidants that fight free radical damage.

In addition, regular fluid intake keeps metabolism active and supports digestion, which are critical elements for a healthy liver. The recipes offered are designed to combine taste and health, offering refreshing and nutritious options that delight the palate and protect the body.

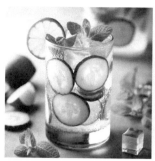

Cucumber Lime Detox Water

Ingredients:
- Sparkling water: 500 ml (16.9 fl)
- Cucumber: ½, thinly sliced
- Lime: 1, squeezed
- Mint leaves: 5-6

Instructions:
- In a pitcher, combine the sparkling water, cucumber slices, lime juice, and mint leaves.
- Mix gently and let sit in the refrigerator for at least 30 minutes to allow the flavors to blend.

Advice:
- Serve over ice for instant refreshment.
- For a stronger flavor, let the detox water sit in the refrigerator for a few hours or overnight.

Health Benefits:
- Cucumber and lime are excellent for hydration and detoxification, helping to cleanse the liver and improve digestion.

Presentation:
- Serve in a tall glass with a slice of lime or cucumber on the rim for an elegant touch.

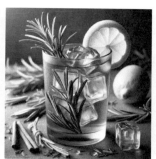

Rosemary and Lemon Iced Tea

Ingredients:
- Black or green tea: 1 liter, (33.8 fl) brewed and chilled
- Fresh rosemary: 1 sprig
- Lemon: 2, the juice and zest
- Honey: 1 tablespoon (optional, for sweetening)

Instructions:
- In a large pitcher, mix the iced tea with the lemon juice and zest.
- Add the rosemary sprig and let it infuse in the refrigerator for at least one hour.

Advice:
- Remove the rosemary sprig after one hour to prevent the flavor from becoming too intense.
- Serve with ice cubes and lemon slices for an added touch of freshness.

Health Benefits:
- Rosemary is known for its antioxidant properties and lemon for its ability to support digestion and purify the body.

Presentation:
- Pour the tea into tall glasses, garnishing with a slice of lemon and a small sprig of rosemary for a refined look.

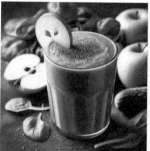

Antioxidant Green Smoothie

Ingredients:
- Fresh spinach: 1 cup, well washed
- Green apple: 1, cut into pieces
- Cucumber: ½, cut into pieces
- Coconut water: 200 ml (6.8 fl)
- Lemon juice: 1 tablespoon
- Chia seeds: 1 teaspoon

Instructions:
- In a blender, add spinach, green apple, cucumber, coconut water, lemon juice and chia seeds.
- Blend at high speed until smooth and homogeneous.

Advice:
- Add a small piece of fresh ginger for a spicy touch that contrasts the sweetness of the apple.
- Serve immediately to preserve the antioxidant properties of the ingredients.

Health Benefits:
- The ingredients in this smoothie are rich in antioxidants, which are essential for fighting free radical damage and supporting the immune system

Presentation:
- Pour the smoothie into a tall glass and, if desired, garnish with a slice of green apple or some extra chia seeds.

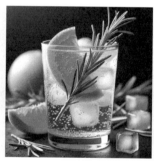

Grapefruit and Rosemary Soda

Ingredients:
- Sparkling water: 500 ml (16.9 fl)
- Grapefruit: 1, squeezed and the zest
- Fresh rosemary: 1 sprig
- Stevia: 1 teaspoon (optional, for sweetening)

Instructions:
- In a glass or pitcher, combine grapefruit juice and stevia.
- Add the sparkling water and stir gently.
- Add the rosemary sprig and let it sit for 10 minutes to allow the flavors to blend.

Advice:
- For more intense flavor, let the rosemary steep longer.
- Serve over ice and garnish with a grapefruit slice or a sprinkling of zest for an elegant touch.

Health Benefits:
- Grapefruit is rich in vitamin C and antioxidants, while rosemary is known for its digestive and anti-inflammatory properties

Presentation:
- Pour the tea into tall glasses, garnishing with a slice of lemon and a small sprig of rosemary for a refined look.

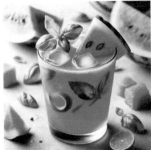

Watermelon and Basil Mocktail

Ingredients:
- Watermelon: 2 cups, diced
- Basil: 10 leaves, plus a few for garnish
- Lime juice: 2 tablespoons
- Sparkling water: 500 ml (16.9 fl)
- Ice: to taste

Instructions:
- In a blender, add the watermelon cubes, lime juice and basil leaves.
- Blend until smooth.
- Pass the liquid through a fine strainer into a pitcher to remove solid residue.
- Add the sparkling water to the strained juice and stir gently.

Advice:
- For a touch of sweetness, you can add some agave syrup or stevia.
- Serve with plenty of ice for a super refreshing mocktail.

Health Benefits:
- Watermelon and basil are rich in antioxidants and vitamins, perfect for hydrating and refreshing the body during the hot months.

Presentation:
- Pour the mocktail into tall glasses, garnishing with a sprinkle of fresh basil leaves and a slice of watermelon.

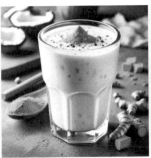

Coconut and Turmeric Lassi

Ingredients:
- Greek yogurt: 200 ml (6.8 fl)
- Coconut milk: 100 ml (3.4 fl)
- Turmeric powder: 1 teaspoon
- Honey: 1 tablespoon
- Black pepper: a pinch (helps the absorption of turmeric)
- Ice: to taste

Instructions:
- In a blender, combine Greek yogurt, coconut milk, turmeric, honey and black pepper.
- Blend until smooth and creamy.
- Add ice and whisk again until the lassi becomes cool and frothy.

Advice:
- You can add some fresh ginger for a spicy touch that complements the sweetness of the honey and the creaminess of the coconut.
- Serve immediately to enjoy the maximum freshness and beneficial properties of turmeric.

Health Benefits:
- Turmeric is known for its anti-inflammatory and antioxidant properties, while coconut provides an excellent source of healthy fats.

Presentation:
- Pour the lassi into tall glasses and garnish with a sprinkling of turmeric or grated coconut for an elegant visual effect.

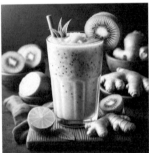

Kiwi and Ginger Smoothie

Ingredients:
- Kiwis: 2, peeled and cut into pieces
- Fresh ginger: 1 cm, peeled and chopped
- Lime juice: 2 tablespoons
- Coconut water: 200 ml (6.8 fl)
- Honey: 1 teaspoon (optional, for sweetening) - Ice to taste

Instructions:
- In a blender, combine the kiwi pieces, chopped ginger, lime juice, coconut water and honey.
- Blend until smooth and creamy.
- Add ice and blend again until the smoothie becomes cool and frothy.

Advice:
- Add a mint or basil leaf for an extra touch of freshness.
- Serve immediately to enjoy all the nutritional benefits and fresh flavor of the smoothie.

Health Benefits:
- Kiwi and ginger are powerful sources of antioxidants and have digestive properties. Kiwi is also rich in vitamin C.

Presentation:
- Pour the smoothie into a tall glass and, if desired, garnish with a slice of green apple or some extra chia seeds.

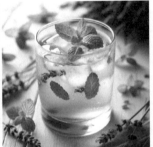

Lavender and Mint Tea

Ingredients:
- Lavender tea: 500 ml, (16.9 fl) brewed and chilled
- Fresh mint leaves: 8-10, plus a few for garnish
- Honey: 1 tablespoon (optional, for sweetening)
- Ice: to taste

Instructions:
- In a pitcher, combine cooled lavender tea with mint leaves.
- Let stand for 10 to 15 minutes to allow the flavors to infuse.
- Remove the mint leaves and sweeten with honey, if desired.

Advice:
- For an even more refreshing flavor, add a few slices of cucumber or lemon to the tea while brewing.
- Serve with plenty of ice to keep the tea fresh and inviting.

Health Benefits:
- Lavender is valued for its calming and relaxing properties, while mint stimulates digestion and refreshes.

Presentation:
- Pour the tea into tall glasses, garnishing with a slice of lemon and a small sprig of rosemary for a refined look.

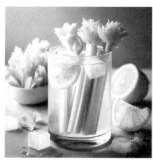

Celery Lemon Flavored Water

Ingredients:
- Water: 1 liter (33.8 fl)
- Celery: 3 stalks, cut into pieces
- Lemon: 1, cut into slices
- Ice: to taste

Instructions:
- In a large pitcher, add the celery pieces and lemon slices.
- Fill it with water and let it infuse in the refrigerator for at least 2-3 hours.
- To serve, add ice and stir gently.

Advice:
- For more intense flavor, lightly mash the celery and lemon before adding them to the water.
- This drink is great for hydration and can be consumed throughout the day.

Health Benefits:
- Celery is known for its diuretic properties that help eliminate toxins, while lemon supports digestion and refreshes.

Presentation:
- Serve this flavored water in clear glasses to show off the celery pieces and lemon slices, making it visually appealing.

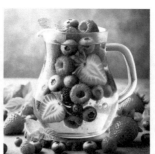

Infusion of Water and Berries

Ingredients:
- Water: 1 liter
- Blueberries: ¼ cup
- Raspberries: ¼ cup
- Strawberries: ¼ cup, cut in half
- Mint leaves: for garnish (optional)

Instructions:
- In a large pitcher, add the blueberries, raspberries and strawberries.
- Pour the water over the fruit and stir gently.
- Let infuse in the refrigerator for at least 4 hours, or overnight to intensify the flavors.

Advice:
- Lightly crush the berries before adding them to the water to release more flavor.
- Add fresh mint leaves before serving for an added touch of freshness.

Health Benefits:
- This infusion is rich in antioxidants thanks to the berries, perfect for hydrating the body and fighting free radicals.

Presentation:
- Serve the infused water in clear glasses to show off the bright colors of the fruit, with a few mint leaves as decoration..

CONCLUSION

Congratulations on completing this cookbook dedicated to liver health. You've taken a vital step towards a healthier life. Managing fatty liver is more than just diet; it's about embracing a healthier lifestyle.
Key Takeaways:

- Balanced Nutrition: A variety of nutrient-rich foods is crucial. While no single food can cure fatty liver, a balanced diet significantly improves liver health.
- Regular Exercise: Aim for at least 30 minutes of activity daily to manage and improve fatty liver.
  Stress Management: Use mindfulness, yoga, and deep breathing to reduce stress, which can affect liver health.
- Consistency: Small, consistent efforts lead to significant improvements over time.

You now have the tools to support your liver through diet and lifestyle changes. The recipes and meal plans are designed to be both delicious and beneficial.
Looking Ahead:

Continue exploring new recipes, staying active, and prioritizing your health. Share your journey with loved ones and seek support when needed. Your dedication is an investment in a brighter future.

Explore more health resources in Mark Ratoy's other books. Each book provides practical tools and knowledge for better health.

If you found this book helpful, follow my upcoming health books. Together, we can make a difference in your life.

With dedication and appreciation,

Mark Ratoy

ACCESS YOUR EXCLUSIVE BONUSES

Thank you for purchasing "The Super Easy Fatty Liver Diet Cookbook"! We are excited to offer you 4 exclusive bonuses to support you on your journey to better liver health. These bonuses include:

- Weekly Meal Planning
- The Fatty Liver Sleep Solution
- Mindful Eating Guide
- Progress Tracking

To download your bonuses, simply scan the QR code below. It's quick and easy!

Instructions below the QR code:

How to Download Your Bonuses:

1. Scan the QR code with your smartphone camera or a dedicated QR code scanning app.
2. Follow the link that will automatically open on your device.
3. Enter your name and email address on the landing page.
4. Download your bonuses directly from the landing page.

Made in the USA
Columbia, SC
20 December 2024

50334296R00046